Mental Health User Narratives

Mental Health User Narratives

New Perspectives on Illness and Recovery

Bruce MZ Cohen
Humboldt Universität zu Berlin

palgrave
macmillan

Softcover reprint of the hardcover 1st edition 2008 978-1-4039-4536-5

First published 2008 by
PALGRAVE MACMILLAN

Palgrave Macmillan in the UK is an imprint of Macmillan Publishers Limited, registered in England, company number 785998, of Houndmills, Basingstoke, Hampshire RG21 6XS.

Palgrave Macmillan in the US is a division of St Martin's Press LLC, 175 Fifth Avenue, New York, NY 10010.

Palgrave Macmillan is the global academic imprint of the above companies and has companies and representatives throughout the world.

Palgrave® and Macmillan® are registered trademarks in the United States, the United Kingdom, Europe and other countries.

ISBN 978-1-349-52297-2 ISBN 978-0-230-59396-1 (eBook)
DOI 10.1057/9780230593961

This book is printed on paper suitable for recycling and made from fully managed and sustained forest sources. Logging, pulping and manufacturing processes are expected to conform to the environmental regulations of the country of origin.

A catalogue record for this book is available from the British Library.

This book is dedicated to all those who have experienced mental health problems.

This is just the beginning of the story.

Contents

List of Tables

Preface

Many studies in the field of mental health have focused on service users as passive recipients of psychiatric care. Assumptions have been made that users are unable of understanding their own illness behaviour. Narrative work within medicine and the social sciences, however, calls for a reassessment of the way we research mental health users, arguing that users are active participants and experts on their own state of being. This book details one of the first studies in the United Kingdom to give primacy to user narratives. The book focuses on the listening to and understanding of the voice of users who have suffered from severe mental illness. It differs from other texts in the field by arguing for the avoidance of immediate interpretation. Instead, user 'narratives' (or stories) are taken at face value, building a more rounded picture of the lives of users, and producing new perspectives on mental health and illness. Insights are gained into such areas as spiritualism, self-coping, self-recovery, alternative treatments, positive illness experience and future life paths. Further, comparison of institutional and 'home treatment' user narratives will illustrate the fluidity of illness identity depending on the psychiatric intervention experienced. Far from severe mental illness being a life sentence, it will be shown that with the right philosophy of care, long-term recovery is possible.

The research in this book will demonstrate a need to widen the therapeutic mind to include the mundane and everyday as an additional focus for treatment. This book is the first volume allowing mental health users to speak to the professional community which offers to treat them and as such will be an important resource for professionals, students and policy makers as well as users and carers in the mental health field.

Acknowledgements

For aiding the funding and progression of the research cited in this book I would like to thank the Bradford Community Health NHS Trust, the University of Bradford's Ethnicity & Social Policy Research Unit, the Bradford Health Authority and the Bradford Home Treatment Service. Research and technical support was provided by Ghazala Mir (bilingual interviews), AC Consultants (transcription), Netta Hollins (hospital databases), the Bradford Community Health NHS Trust's Information Section, the University of Bradford Computer Centre and the Department of Social and Economic Studies's administrative staff (especially Jane Hammond).

For advice, support and encouragement with the original study I would to thank my colleagues in Bradford: Ian Burkitt, Charles Husband, Rampaul Chamba, Apurba Kundu, Stacey Burlet, Yunas Samad and Stephen Collins. Colin Samson at the University of Essex was also a decent chap. Thanks also to Pat Bracken, Phil Thomas and all the Bradford Home Treatment Service staff for being friendly and helpful, yet not interfering with the research.

For facilitating the development of the book I would like to thank Sabine Michalowski. For the useful conversations on developments in the UK health system, I thank David Cohen, Val Rhodes, Neil Brimblecombe, Lizzie Cohen and Gill Rowe-Aslam. Hilary Lapsley and her research on user narratives in New Zealand was also inspirational. Thank you also to Palgrave and my editor, Jill Lake, for support and amazing patience. On a personal note, thanks to friends and family in Berlin and the United Kingdom, especially Jessica Terruhn, Hadischa and Fanelli.

Finally, heartfelt thanks to all the mental health users who allowed me to listen to their stories.

List of Abbreviations

BHTS	Bradford Home Treatment Service
BMJ	British Medical Journal
CMHRC	Community Mental Health Resource Centre
CPN	Community Psychiatric Nurse
CRT	Crisis Resolution Team
CTO	Community Treatment Order
DLP	Daily Living Programme (Maudsley)
DSM	Diagnostic and Statistical Manual of Mental Disorders
ECT	Electroconvulsive Therapy
EU	European Union
GP	General Practitioner
ICD	International Classification of Diseases
NHS	National Health Service
NUD.IST	Non-Numerical Unstructured Data Indexing Searching and Theory Building
RMO	Responsible Medical Officer
SMI	Severe Mental Illness
UK	United Kingdom
US	United States

Introduction

The World Health Organization (2005a) estimates that 450 million people worldwide currently experience 'mental, neurological or behavioural problems'. In the United States alone, almost 44 million people – approximately one in six of the population – are affected by a mental illness in any given year (United States Department of Health and Human Services 2002). Likewise, the Office for National Statistics (2001: 1) calculates that, at any one time, one in six of the UK population experiences a 'significant' mental health problem. The European Union, meanwhile, suggests that mental ill health affects one in four of their citizens (European Commission Health and Consumer Protection Directorate-General 2005: 3). On the basis of such figures it is accurate to comment that, sooner or later, most of us will experience some form of mental illness: it is an illness of the majority not the minority. Despite mental illness being responsible for approximately 13 per cent of all disease burden in the world and ranking 'first among illnesses that cause disability in the United States, Canada, and Western Europe' (President's New Freedom Commission on Mental Health 2003: 3), most countries continue to give a low priority to mental health care (World Health Organization 2005b). The costs of mental illness to society are enormous: in the United States, the indirect costs (loss of productivity and so on) are estimated to be in the region of $79 billion per annum whilst a further $71 billion per annum is spent on treatment (President's New Freedom Commission on Mental Health 2003: 3).

But what exactly is 'mental illness'? What does it mean to have a mental health problem? Over the past few centuries the nature and form of mental illness in Western society has been widely debated, different theories have been proffered, different treatments developed and, thus, different 'cures' for illness claimed. Mountains of literature have been published on the subject – from moral therapy through the development of new biochemical compounds for treatment to detailing life in psychiatric hospitals. And yet at the beginning of the 21st century, how far can we say we have come in successfully defining and understanding what mental illness actually is? Of course, we have successfully developed groups of experts and practitioners who claim to know what mental illness is and how we can avoid it in our everyday lives. But if you are a mental health practitioner, a service user, a carer or even a researcher you may still be left wondering why the theories of mental health do not match with your own experiences of having or working with someone with mental health problems. This is the central objective of the book: to explore mental illness and what it might consist of. To do this we have to temporarily suspend our own (often professional) beliefs. We need to take at face value what we see and hear from the one source that lies at the heart of the mental health debate but is often ignored – from the service users themselves.

Through reproduction and further analysis of 49 user narratives, this book explores the descent into illness, experiences of institutional psychiatry and home treatment, patterns of recovery and self-coping techniques. The book embeds the reader in the life worlds of those who have suffered mental health problems. There is no finite solution offered, no silver bullet for these problems in living, but the book highlights new approaches to such illnesses and new ways of recovery. The title of this book is as much a political statement as a scientific claim because it challenges the dominant wisdom within psychiatry that users understand very little about their own problems. The 'narrative method' used in this research empowers the user and asks us to think again about the personal nature of illness experience.

Most people diagnosed with a mental health problem will not require specialist psychiatric services (see MIND 2005). In contrast, this book reproduces the narratives of those who have suffered from a 'severe mental illness' (SMI). An SMI is a mental illness that usually requires a period of hospitalization. The President's New Freedom Commission on Mental Health (2003: 2) estimates that between five and seven per cent of all adults in the United States have a severe mental illness (such as schizophrenia or manic depression) in any given year. These SMIs cause the largest economic and social burden on society because they are the most incapacitating of mental illnesses. In the past, those suffering from an SMI required long-term institutional care, yet new medical treatments combined with crisis intervention projects and deinstitutionalization policies have suggested that many can survive without the need for in-patient treatment. In realty, the problem of how to treat this small but highly significant population of users has never been fully resolved. Governmental reviews of mental health policy in Europe and the United States raise similar questions about the uneven base of mental health care, levels of stigmatization, the need for treatment close to home and so on, but provide less tangible solutions (for example, Department of Health 1999, 2007; European Commission Health and Consumer Protection Directorate-General 2005; Jané-Llopis and Anderson 2005; President's New Freedom Commission on Mental Health 2003). In the 21st century, the neo-liberalist concepts of choice, customer care and quality of service are tempered in mental health by the factor of risk – those suffering from SMIs are perceived as being a threat to the public as well as to themselves (Department of Health 1999, 2007; McLaughlin 2006; MIND 2007a). In such cases, mental health policy allows for compulsory medical treatment as well as compulsory hospital admittance. This is sometimes seen as the 'balanced system of care' (Thornicroft and Tansella 2004) in which both hospital and community services are necessary for mental health users. Through comparison of two forms of acute care – hospitalization and home treatment – for those suffering from SMIs this book also assesses the possibility of treating the most severe mental illnesses without the need for institutional treatment.

To summarize then, this book has three main aims: firstly, to investigate periods of mental illness for those defined as acute or severe mental health users with reference to their life stories (or 'narratives'); secondly, to demonstrate the possibility of taking a 'narrative approach' within research methodology and analysis; and, thirdly, to compare the narratives of users who have obtained hospital-only treatment with users who received a new home treatment service. The book is divided into two parts – the first part grounds the reader in the debates on mental illness, narrative theory, crisis intervention projects and narrative methodology; the second part reproduces the user narratives and offers further analysis of these texts. Much of the first half is unapologetically theoretical, for those who wish to move straight to the narratives I would recommend starting at Chapter 5. Additionally, one piece of text from a user narrative is given at the start of each chapter.

An investigation of mental illness experience necessarily involves an investigation of the history and current status of psychiatry. Chapter 1 profiles the rise of psychiatric professionals as the medical experts chiefly responsible for the care of the mentally ill. Whilst producing a dominant medical aetiology with which to understand mental illness, it will be demonstrated that this premise has been constantly critiqued from both inside and outside the profession. A discussion of critical psychiatry will highlight the current views towards psychiatric treatment within the field – psychiatrists often perceive their treatment methods with users as pragmatic and eclectic, yet medical treatment (that is, drugs or ECT) remains omnipresent.

Disillusionment with traditional modes of treatment has led some psychiatrists to take a 'narrative approach' with users. Within psychiatry this approach is seen as a way of changing the balance of power between psychiatrist and user. Chapter 2 introduces the reader to the 'narrative' concept. Critiques of modernity and traditional scientific practice have led to the proliferation of 'narrative approaches' not only within psychiatry, psychology and the therapeutic disciplines but also in the humanities and social sciences. Different definitions and uses which surround this move to narrative are outlined before describing an appropriate theoretical background and definition used in the current research with mental health users.

Crisis intervention projects hold an important place within the development of community-based psychiatric care because they have often attempted to prevent hospitalization for those experiencing an acute crisis. Chapter 3 describes the development of crisis theory and the introduction of crisis intervention projects such as home treatment services. Some time is spent surveying the background, philosophy and development of a home treatment project in Bradford, United Kingdom, which explicitly sought to work with a needs-led approach to psychiatric treatment for those suffering from an SMI. The investigation of this Bradford Home Treatment Service gives the reader a good example of a successful alterative to hospital care that nevertheless suffered changes in its workings due to changing governmental policy. The benefits of this crisis intervention service to local mental health users will be witnessed in the chapters that follow.

A practical account of taking the 'narrative method' in the current research with mental health users is outlined in Chapter 4. Sampling and collection procedures for both hospital and home treatment users are described. Some time is also spent detailing the piloting and introduction of the narrative approach. The problems of the method, particularly regarding the analysis and presentation of the texts, are discussed in detail. Whilst being able to offer some generalizations of user experience, the concern to avoid interpretation of the user narratives results in the different methods of text reproduction outlined in Chapters 5, 6 and 7.

Eight of the user narratives collected – four who experienced home treatment and four who were hospitalized – are reproduced, as close to the original texts as possible, in Chapter 5. It is necessarily the longest chapter in the book, recounting significant life stories of the mental health users. The narratives from those who have experienced hospital treatment tend to concentrate more on illness feelings and psychiatric treatment whilst the home treatment narratives are often broader, illustrating a life that is not always defined by severe mental illness and treatment. Yet the narratives remain fluid and multifaceted, calling for some further analysis of all 49 life stories.

The descent into illness and the periods of psychiatric treatment cited in the user narratives are explored in Chapter 6. Precipitating factors to crisis and referral processes are given, before a detailed analysis of both hospital and home treatment are carried out. Both treatment options are assessed on the basis of user narratives, and improvements are outlined. The narratives highlight the value of the home treatment service and its innovative philosophy, whilst hospitalization also has a number of benefits for some. In both cases, the user narrative is altered by the professional, psychiatric narrative.

The recovery from illness and self-coping strategies are outlined in Chapter 7. A number of significant issues – not often cited in books on mental illness – are highlighted here including the routes out of illness, surviving without psychiatric treatment and user methods of coping with crises. As periods of illness come to be perceived in different ways, so too do ways of self-coping in day-to-day life. It is shown that some service users can alter their illness label downwards, from a severe mental illness to a milder form of mental illness, and in doing so create their own possibilities for recovery. Personal meanings of illness call for personal solutions. Everyday practices – such as work, socializing, sleeping and shopping – are highlighted as significant therapeutic activities for users.

In Chapter 8, the book concludes with a reiteration of the intentions of reproducing the narratives of mental health users. Time is given to explore the workings of the psychiatric paradigm as outlined by the users themselves. Factors of gender, ethnicity and social class in treatment are also summarized. The rest of the chapter offers a discussion of the dominant psychiatric view of mental illness and appropriate treatment in comparison to users' own experiences of illness and recovery. Implications for the future are highlighted in the concluding remarks.

1
Mental Illness and Psychiatry

> 'Manic depression' and... labeled as a 'schizophrenic', 'paranoid schizophrenic' at one point in time. But, you know, the classic question is, they ask you, is, 'do you hear voices?' you know, 'when you're on your own?' sort of thing... and only my own. But I don't hear voices, I just don't.
>
> (Bill)

1.1 Summary

This book unashamedly gives primacy to those who have experienced severe or acute periods of mental ill health. The narratives from these users will offer new insights into illness and recovery. Over 30 years ago, Mosher *et al.* (1975: 455–6) asked the rhetorical question, 'who can tell us better how to get over the illness than its recovered victims?' It was not the first time – nor the last – that the suggestion was made for the centrality of the voice of the user in understanding mental illness. Yet in 2007, this book is one of the first to comprehensively investigate user narratives without the interception of medical or psychological interpretation. This begs the question as to why it has taken us so long to get to this position. Why has the voice of the service user been marginalized? To answer this question it is necessary to briefly survey the history of madness, the development of the mental health field as a medical project and the rise of psychiatry as the profession chiefly responsible for the care and treatment of the mentally ill. It will be shown that psychiatry is not only a medical project but also a political one. Despite conflicting views on the definition and nature of mental illness within the profession – leading to a variety of treatment options – medical intervention continues unabated, encouraged by the pharmaceutical industry. The result is a continued devaluing and disempowerment of user meanings for illness.

1.2 Histories of madness

1.2.1 The official account

The 'official account' of psychiatry's history, as often profiled in medical text books, is one of slow but steady progress from the unenlightened days of the mistreatment of lunatics in places like Bedlam to the present state of medical expertise (Johnstone 1989). Three key phases are cited in the official account of this progression. Firstly, the shift in the 19th century from primitive views of madness as caused by supernatural agencies to a more sophisticated medical view, with the era of 'moral treatment' ending the worse excesses. Secondly, the development of some local outpatients and aftercare facilities in the 1930s, as well as the discovery of new treatments such as insulin coma therapy and electroconvulsive therapy (ECT). Thirdly, the 'drug revolution' of the 1950s which enabled discharge and the possibility of users living outside of the psychiatric hospital. Thus, psychiatry becomes accepted as part of the medical establishment and patients avoid the stigma of the old asylums by attending psychiatric units at general hospitals (Johnstone 1989: 172–3).

The history of madness and psychiatry that I will outline challenges this official account, highlighting social, economic and political processes in the identification and treatment of those considered 'mad'. As Miller (1986: 13) has stated, 'the history of psychiatry is a history of fundamental transformations of its institutional, theoretical, professional and judicial existence. The critiques mounted against psychiatry, both from inside and outside, are a significant element in this process of modernization and transformation'.

1.2.2 Pre-psychiatric care

'Prior to the mid-17th century and the advent of the "Classical Age" ', states Smart (1985: 2), 'madness or unreason and reason itself were relatively integrated phenomena'. 'Madness' could be associated with special, sacred forms of knowledge which gave insights into the human condition. The insane were not stigmatized or removed from the community in which they lived; instead they were an active part of communal life. Kosky (1986), for example, notes that during the 16th century the insane were mainly cared for by relatives. Additionally, medical practitioners were present in most villages and provided an eclectic approach to madness which could involve utilizing diets, laxatives, baths, exercises, purgatives and blood-letting. In cases of suspected depossessions, clerics were called to deal with evil spirits. The medical practitioners themselves were trained by apprenticeship and licensed by the church through bishops. In the cases of the more difficult 'insane', hospitals (such as St Bartholomew's established in 1123 and Bethlem established in 1250) accepted such people on a short- or long-term basis. Taxes were levied on parishes to supplement families caring for insane relatives or for help with hospital fees, and peoples' property was protected by royal prerogatives or Court of Wards (Kosky 1986: 180–1). Kosky acknowledges that 'there are accounts of the insane being imprisoned, held in stocks, whipped and driven from village to village. Nevertheless, the 16th century bore witness to a relatively tolerant and humanistic attitude to the mad and to mental illness' (1986: 181). Likewise, Samson (1995b: 56) notes that although punishment – including the gallows and burning at the stake – existed for the mad it was far from systematic.

In these years before the Enlightenment lunatics were often treated by the family, the clergy, the jailer, the workhouse master and the magistrate rather than by medical men (Scull 1981b). Most importantly though, what was seen as 'teachings of madness' could take a variety of forms and supposed 'cures' during the period. 'Madness' was not attached to the idea of 'moral value' (see also Kroll and Bachrach 1984); that is, there was no separation between the spiritual and the material worlds of the time. People were not conceptualized as *individually conscious* of their own behaviour and thought. Morality was a collective process of the whole society given through religious and monarchical authorities from God. As a result of the explosion of new ideas taking place towards the end of the 16th and into the 17th centuries, however, inevitable upheavals were about to take place in the realm of the spirit (Zweig 1979). Medical practitioners had already made successful moves to separate from the church and establish their independence as professionals with primacy in medical matters. A few London- or university-based doctors of classically derived medicine established the Foundation of London Society of Physicians in 1518 and by the end of the century the group had hounded out even the popular bishop-licensed medical practitioners.

1.2.3 The Enlightenment

Bracken and Thomas (2001) note that 'both supporters and critics of psychiatry agree that the discipline is a product of the European

Enlightenment and that movement's preoccupations with reason and the individual subject'. The Enlightenment brought about far-reaching changes in Western society: the separation of the individual from society, man from God, a move towards secularization and the explosion of ideas initiated by philosophers such as Descartes and Newton, which led to the observable and measurable universe of science. Freeman (1996) locates the philosophical basis of psychiatry in the work of Hobbes (1588–1679) and Locke (1632–1704), both of whom were empiricists and rejected the notion of any *a priori* knowledge existing in the mind; instead peoples' knowledge was derived from experience of the world. Envisaging man as an individual, Hobbes proclaimed, 'the succession of our thoughts is not arbitrary, but governed by laws' (cited in Russell 1984: 533). All men were naturally equal – 'in a state of nature' – but without a social contract to bind people together in communities and to the state (and thus to control their natural state), life would be 'nasty, short, and brutal'. Hobbes's concern was for society to maintain a consensus and some form of control over people's autonomy, whilst Locke's 'philosophical liberalism' argued for the pursuit of happiness as the foundation of all freedom (Russell 1984: 592). What psychiatry took from these ideas were a mixture of liberalism, empiricism and the control of people's 'natural state'.

Kosky believes these new philosophies were also tied to Calvinistic ideas: non-conformity was not only an affront to God; it was also representing subversion of the state. Numbers of the so-called deviant classes (the heretics, criminals, unemployed, sexually deviant, socially rebellious and the insane) had greatly increased due to the long religious wars in Europe and 'concern for organization and order under these conditions focused attention of authorities, secular and religious, on these classes' (Kosky 1986: 181). The stage was set for what Foucault calls 'the great confinement' of these undesirable classes in Western Europe. Foucault has argued in his book *Madness and Civilisation* (1967) that structures of exclusion and division had been dormant since the existence of leprosy in Europe in the Middle Ages and were ready to return with the new period of incarceration in the 17th and 18th centuries; 'when the poor, criminals, and those with "deranged minds" were compelled to occupy the space of exclusion which had been vacated by the leper' (Smart 1985: 3).

Scull (1981b: 113) contends that it was the changes brought about by growing market forces and industrialization that fundamentally changed popular conceptions of human nature: 'economic competition and the factory system are the forcing house for a thoroughgoing transformation in the relation of man to man'. Industrial capitalism demanded a reform of character on the part of men and women (see Pollard 1965, cited in Scull 1981b), and an internalization of these new norms. There was a growing sense that men and women were masters of their own destinies. The old ideas of 'the suppression of evil' or 'the breaking of the will' were outdated to the new mode of production and were replaced by the possibility that people could change and improve – an idea of the *reform* of one's own character. Thus, Locke's concept of reward and punishment brought about changes in the 18th century from the idea of crime being innate and immovably wicked or sinful, to the ranks of common humanity where other factors such as social and economic conditions could be seen to play an important part in the moral condition of citizens. These people still had *reason* in common with other people and, accordingly, they could be 're-moulded' from such a 'defective mechanism' (see Scull 1981b: 114). Likewise, if the individual was in a state of irrational behaviour and thought, they could also become rational beings again through the reformation of character. Thus, the idea of a 'fixed' human under the gaze of a deity had changed to one of the flexible individual who had the power to change and grow.

Between the Renaissance and the end of the 19th century two conceptions replaced the pre-Enlightenment idea of the mad. Firstly, certain patterns of behaviour and mental states became the result of *disease*; thus the proper object of medical description was *treatment*. Secondly, *the mind became a function of the brain*. These physical and mental processes were so closely linked that one could not be properly understood without reference to the other (Bynum 1981: 35). A new arm of medicine – psychiatry – developed during this period to act as the appropriate experts on madness. The discipline was actually a by-product of the institutionalization of the 'insane'.

1.2.4 The great confinement

Institutions for the criminal, the poor, the sick and the insane sprang up across much of Europe as the Enlightenment gathered speed and industrialization began. By the mid-18th century, institutions for the mentally ill had been established in many British cities (Freeman 1996). Scull (1981a) notes the Victorian pride and complacency in their response to the mentally ill. A partial history of madness was emphasized at this time: insane people had been treated with cruelty and subjected to various inhumane practices in the past but were now treated in a moral and humanitarian fashion. In many quarters the new 'moral treatment' of the insane was also viewed as scientific, 'an interpretation those segments of the medical profession that were involved in the treatment of lunacy were initially very keen to promulgate' (Scull 1981a: 1). The institutions were overseen by 'medical superintendents of asylums for the insane', and Scull (1981a: 6) sees this title as evidence of the clumsiness of the emerging professional identity of psychiatry, bound up as it was with their institutional status. Henceforth, 'the character and course of mental illness [were to be] ... shaped irrevocably by medical intervention' (Sedgwick 1982: 128).

With the growth of the institutions for 'the mad', Scull believes the medical profession was able to change the somatic disorder, claiming that *both* medical and moral treatment was essential for the treatment of mental illness. The Victorian age witnessed 'the transformation of the madhouse into the asylum into the mental hospital; of the mad-doctor into the alienist into the psychiatrist; and of the madman (and madwoman) into the mental patient' (Scull 1981a: 6). The era saw dramatic changes in society's response to madness: the state apparatus assumed a much greater role, asylums became almost the sole official response to problems of the mentally disordered, and the nature and limits of lunacy were themselves transformed.

Though moral treatment and the rise of state-sponsored asylums were meant to emphasize the care and curability of the insane, the buildings followed designs similar to Victorian prisons, suggesting the continuing idea of constraint and the improbability of the insane person regaining reason (Scull 1981a: 9). Scull comments that the institutions were,

> The almost exclusive arena in which the new profession [psychiatry] plied its trade. The structure of moral treatment was such that the asylum was also perceived by alienists as one of their crucial therapeutic instruments; that is, the asylum itself was a major weapon (perhaps *the* major weapon) in the struggle to cure the insane.
>
> (1981a: 9, emphasis original)

Thus, ideological justification for the expertise of the alienists was achieved by stressing an exclusive experience of running the asylums and the positive benefits of asylum treatment. Asylum reformers both in Britain and in the United States had an unshakeable conviction that lunacy was curable, even if 'asylums increasingly degenerated into little more than custodial warehouses' (Scull 1981a: 12). Eventually, advocates for the institutions began to argue for extending these 'benefits' to those – particularly the more 'respectable' elements of society – who would not use the asylum's services. It was the start of psychiatry's transformation from a purely institutional-based profession.

1.2.5 Deinstitutionalization

For a hundred years, up until the 1950s, most Western societies witnessed large increases in the number of asylums and the annual population in each asylum. Scull (1984: 67) notes that in Britain in 1850 there were 7140 people in public asylums (4.03 per 10,000 of population), yet by 1954 there were 148,000 people (33.45 per 10,000 of population) in such institutions. Since 1954, however, there have been year-on-year decreases in that population. The 1950s marked the beginning of a 'revolution' in psychiatric treatment which aided explanations for the decline in the hospital population as well as the accelerated rate of discharge. Scull (1984: 79) comments,

> At the very least, one must acknowledge that in this period [psychiatrists] were given a new treatment modality which enabled them to engage in a more passable imitation of conventional medical practice. In place of acting as glorified administrators of huge custodial warehouses, and instead of relying on crude empirical devices like shock therapy and even cruder surgical techniques like lobotomy to provide themselves with an all too transparent medical figleaf, psychiatrists in public mental hospitals could now engage in the prescription and administration of the classic symbolic accoutrement of the modern medicine man – drugs.

The psychiatric profession claimed that the introduction of new pharmaceutical technologies and a corresponding increase in 'curability' rates were responsible for the decline in hospital populations. Drugs were seen as a far more effective and cheaper way of treating psychiatric patients (by 1970, pharmaceutical manufacturers had sold $500 million of 'psychotherapeutic agents' in the United States alone). But this is an inaccurate conclusion. In the United Kingdom, for example, hospital populations were in decline *before* the introduction of such drugs. The number of *admissions*, however, continued to increase after this period despite the decline in the overall population, suggesting a 'policy of greater accelerated discharging' (Scull 1984: 67). The 'cult of curability' era – which had marked the beginning of the psychiatric profession – had subsequently been dropped in favour of rapid diagnosis, treatment and discharge. Scull concludes that the institutions seemed 'largely unconcerned with labelling their output as cured' (1984: 67).

Scull suggests that, at best, psychotropic drugs may have assisted in early discharges by calming some of the symptoms of mental illness. On the whole, the effect of the introduction of drugs has been exaggerated and cannot give feasibility to the universal 'deinstitutionalization' policy which followed. 'Deinstitutionalization' is described by Scull (1984: 1) as,

> Shorthand for a state-sponsored policy of closing down asylums, prisons and reformatories. Mad people, criminals, and delinquents are being discharged or refused admissions to the dumps in which they have been traditionally housed. Instead, they are to be left at large, to be coped with 'in the community'.

In both the United States and the United Kingdom in the mid-1950s it became apparent that there were still bed shortages as well as a need for very expensive repairs to the large Victorian asylums. What has been described as a more 'humane' way of caring for people within their local environment is seen by Scull and others as a rhetorical justification for the wholesale closure of large and expensive institutions and the provision of a cheaper form of 'care in the community'. Scull (1984) points to the inevitability of community care as a result of the 'success' of 20th century welfare capitalism. By the 1970s, commentators had become quite blunt about the economic realties of the mental health system. Greenblatt (1974) commented, 'in a sense our backs are to the wall; it's *phase out* before we go *bankrupt*', while Dingman (1974) added that 'rising costs more than any other factor have made it obvious that support of state hospitals is politically unfeasible... this is the principal factor behind the present push to get rid of state hospitals' (both cited in Scull 1984: 139, emphases original).

Although the United Kingdom had particular ideological as well as economic reasons for closing down public hospitals, Scull notes that the arguments put forward against mental hospital treatment in the 20th century were fairly similar to those put forward by some observers in the 19th century. It was the ensuing pressures of the modern welfare state that had changed the situation. As he explains, 'the arguments had not changed, but the structural context in which they were advanced clearly had. Their contemporary reappearance allowed governments to save money while simultaneously giving their policy a humanitarian gloss' (1984: 139).

1.2.6 Community care

Griffiths (1988) has talked of 'community care' as care provided to people 'in their own homes, group homes, residential care homes, hostels and nursing homes' (cited in Prior 1993: 169), the implication being that community care is the opposite of any form of hospital-based care. Prior (1993) notes that in the late 20th century the community came to be regarded as the 'cornerstone' of psychiatry and other forms of medical practice – services were now organized around the community as a matter of routine. But the nature of the 'community' can take many forms and can also be readily found in the hospital: the 'therapeutic community' of the asylum/hospital, for example, or self-help colonies of the 1960s. The 'community' and the hospital have only recently been regarded as separate from one another. Prior follows Miller in citing psychiatry as moving from the 'intramural community' of the insane to the 'extramural community' of people with psychiatric disorders. Following the critique of Morel and others of the institutional basis of psychiatry, more emphasis was placed on the social basis of mental illness. On this basis it became clear that treating and normalizing social relations in an artificial and isolated setting was not conducive to good mental health. Prior also points to psychiatry's expanding diagnoses and increasing number of associated disorders and disturbances; 'lunacy' decreased whilst cases of neuroses and behavioural disorders increased. These disorders were seen as less set apart from everyday behaviour; rather they were only extreme cases of otherwise 'normal' thought and behaviour. When to these factors is added a growing recognition that psychiatric disorders appeared to have a certain social context in which they developed – as well as a certain social distribution – 'we begin to see a suitable mix of reasons as to why the psychiatric and related professions turned their attentions outward beyond the asylum walls and into non-institutional settings' (Prior 1993: 105).

We can see how the last factor impacted on psychiatric thought and practice in the 1960s, a period which Slater and Roth (1969) describe as 'extreme and profound' for psychiatry. With its dominant positivistic philosophy, the revelation that epidemiological studies of the general population showed the 'actual' rate of mental illness in the community to be much greater than the current detection rates (as well as suggesting a mix of social and physiological causes to mental illness) gave the profession justification of what is sometimes felt to be a 'revolution' in psychiatry at the time. Following a widening of medicine's 'clinical gaze' (Armstrong 1983) in the 1920s and 1930s, studies suggested the distribution of mental disturbances in the community were widely underestimated. Following the Second World War, epidemiologists began distinguishing between *incidence rates* (rates of new cases of different mental illnesses) and *prevalence rates* (rates of existing mental illness) in studies of the general population carried out in Europe and North America. Shepherd (1966), for example, estimated that one-fifth of the adult population in the United Kingdom was in need of treatment and that there was a 'reservoir' of cases, far in excess of what present referrals to psychiatrists indicated. A potential prevalence rate of 70 per 1000 was suggested, with the majority of psychiatric patients suffering from minor disorders. These figures were backed up by subsequent studies (for example, Wing *et al.* 1981).

In seeking to measure the prevalence of mental illness, however, one has to question what is meant by the term in the first place, and this has been found to change over the course of the 20th century. Whereas, for instance, Kraepelian psychiatry assumed a physical reality to mental diseases, people such as Szasz (1970) and Sedgwick (1982) questioned the very notion of 'mental illness' and 'normalization', believing the debate to be one about the nature of human reality itself rather than about agreement of terminology. The validity of all the epidemiological surveys were questioned in the 1970s and 1980s, with Bachelard (1984) arguing that such research merely produced the phenomena which it claimed to discover and measure. Despite such critiques, community surveys had the desired effect of undermining the rationale of the isolated and self-controlled psychiatric hospitals, and of establishing the new rationale of community psychiatry.

Though piecemeal, 20th century philosophy also served to undermine the idea of the isolated individual with disorders of the brain. Surveys amongst local populations sought to correlate mental illness with particular socio-economic variables such as occupational group, social class, gender, ethnic group, age group, housing conditions, general level of health, familial status and so on. Durkheim's (1952) study of suicide as a form of insanity in 1897 – which suggested rates of suicide correlated with dominant religious philosophies of a given society – was an early challenge to the idea of humans as simply biologically determined organisms. Faris and Dunham (1939) of the Chicago School were another example: they suggested that mental illness was directly related to social (urban) disorganization. This nature versus nurture debate in mental illness continued throughout the last century and undoubtedly aided psychiatry's transition from the psychiatric hospital to the outside world.

There has been an ongoing debate from inside and outside psychiatry as to the impact of community care on the profession. Some argue that it is a threat to psychiatry's power as the designated 'experts' in the field of mental health, some that it is an effective way of strengthening psychiatry's power base from the hospital into the community, others see it as further (state) social control over people's lives in general, while yet still others argue it is the inevitable result of psychiatry's changes in its internal structures. And on this point theorists do not readily look towards the available evidence for the inter-relation between community care and psychiatry's place within the present mental health system but rather focus on their own ideological viewpoints. Thus, Johnstone (1989) is of the view that the rise of community care is a direct attack on traditional medical model psychiatry and it is these psychiatric workers who are the greatest critics of the legislation, believing it will undermine their position of power as the 'experts' on issues of mental health. 'The crucial question for community care', states Johnstone (1989: 188), 'is whether it will be able to live up to its promise of moving away from traditional medical model-style psychiatry. If not, then it will not have been a change for the better'.

One has to ask if the rhetoric of community care ever included a premise of moving away from 'traditional medical model-style psychiatry' or if it was ever believed by policy makers that this was a strategic part of such social policy change. For as Prior (1993: 176) states, 'the broad thrust of care in the community policies often appear to be driven by political rather than traditional psychiatric concerns'. Banton *et al.* (1985: 165) add that the community cannot be regarded as simply the antithesis of the oppressive and bureaucratic nature of the state and powerful interest groups – that is, the community is in some way inherently progressive. Whilst recognizing that there can be resistance to forces like psychiatry in the community, it is not in itself a radical entity, 'but has a function in the production of ideology and control as well as a potential for resistance – just like any other political space'. This explains why both left-wing and right-wing ideologies can perceive local/community activities as a positive thing. Following this, Bean and Mounser (1993) suggest that, through community care policies, 'social control is being extended to the wider group, the multi-disciplinary team, who are gradually coming to have more and more powers in line with the medical model which they appear to emulate' (1993: 85).

Miller (1986), however, argues that community care is not simply about psychiatry having more effective methods of social control but also about the changing standpoint of psychiatry – as well as new health strategies – to operate across the community rather than in the institution. In contrast, Prior (1993: 125) sees the process of internal struggle within psychiatry and health as secondary to the changes within social policy. He states,

> Perhaps the greatest change of all was truly to be found in the language of social policy rather than in the field of epidemiology: and in particular in a redefinition of the term community so as to exclude its older, religious connotations and to emphasize its geographical and locational ones. Hence, in the new lexicon of the late twentieth century, it became impossible to equate community with asylum, or havens with hospitals. Instead it was taken for granted that the worst home was always superior to the best institution.

1.2.7 Post-community care

Following community care legislation in the early 1990s, Samson (1995a: 265) perceived British psychiatry as being at a 'pivotal juncture', facing fundamental threats to its traditional power base and at the same time resisting these erosions through the assimilation of new practices. Fundamental shifts in the professional power and influence of mental health services in Britain had resulted from Thatcherite health service reforms of the late 1980s and early 1990s. These reforms can be summarized as a move from the hospital to the community, privatization and the contracting out of health care, and a move towards managerial as opposed to medical control. Samson (1995a: 246) stated that,

> Community care, as a conduit for the shift from NHS [National Health Service] provision to private, voluntary and local authority provision through the contracting out process, present fundamental dilemmas for the profession of psychiatry since its status, power and pre-eminent role in treatment has been so closely tied to the authority structures of the NHS.

Traditionally, psychiatrists have been the most powerful group in the mental health field with the perceived expertise to define illness, decide who should be admitted to hospital and prescribe treatment, as well as enforce any administrative and legal powers found necessary for the good of the patient. The profession has also overseen the mental health hierarchies of nursing, social work and psychology. By contrast, community care policy looked outside the National Health Service (NHS) to provide much of the provision and direction. This base of knowledge, which was in many respects non-medical, was a 'potential threat to the traditional leadership and authority of the psychiatrist, and, by extension, to the continued utilization of biomedical discourse upon which legitimacy of the profession has been constructed' (Samson 1995a: 247).

It has been argued, however, that the skills of psychiatrists make them the obvious choice to take the leadership role in community mental health provision (Sims 1989). The psychiatric profession was obviously concerned that community provision would see an undermining of their exclusive authority in mental health treatment, but Samson also suggested that as long as medical treatment remained a high-profile treatment the profession would be ensured continuation, being the only ones who can prescribe drugs and courses of electroconvulsive therapy (ECT). Far from declining in psychiatric treatment, drugs and ECT have in fact continued unabated through the 1980s and 1990s, perpetuated by the myths of quick, cheap and efficient remedies to mental health problems whilst shortening periods of hospital care (see Samson 1995a: 254–8).

In the 1990s, Britain witnessed a number of media-hyped cases that can be dubbed 'scare in the community' (for example, MIND 2006; Muijen 1996; Smith 1997); a string of high-profile assaults against the general public from people diagnosed as mentally ill were quickly attributed to the breakdown of the community care system (Peay 1996). In 1998, the then Minister for Health, Frank Dobson (Department of Health 1998), stated,

> Care in the community has failed. Discharging people from institutions has brought benefits to some. But it has left many vulnerable patients to try to cope on their own. Others have been left to become a danger to themselves and a nuisance to others. Too many confused and sick people have been left wandering the streets and sleeping rough. A small but significant minority have become a danger to the public as well as themselves.

The concepts of 'risk assessment' and 'risk management' were becoming a significant part of post-community care mental health discourse. After a lack of clear 'top-down' guidance from government for the implementation of community care, the Labour government began to lay out plans for the 'modernization' of mental health services (Brimblecombe 2001: 23). The resulting National Service Framework for Mental Health (Department of Health 1999) put an emphasis on caring for those with severe and acute illnesses (SMIs), calling for more acute hospital beds and more crisis intervention teams as well as the enforcement of community treatment orders (CTOs) on those users who were unwilling to take their prescribed medication. The National Service Framework also initiated a comprehensive review of the United Kingdom's mental health legislation (largely based on the Mental Health Act 1983), which ended in March 2006 with the abandonment of the new Mental Health Bill after it had been attacked by both professional and user groups as 'draconian' (for example, James 2006). By the end of the year, the British government had introduced another Mental Health Bill to extend powers of compulsory detention and treatment over people diagnosed with a mental illness through revisions to the Mental Health Act 1983 (see McLaughlin 2006). Meanwhile, both the EU and the United States have also been involved in reviews of care for people suffering mental health problems (see European Commission Health and Consumer Protection Directorate-General 2005; Jané-Llopis and Anderson 2005; President's New Freedom Commission on Mental Health 2003). Thus, the current post-community care mindset is one of review; this includes a reassessment of the infrastructure of mental health services, expansion of crisis intervention and outreach services, the reasserting of a need for some sort of institutional care, a concern with public safety and a need to confront the stigmatization of mental illness. As a result, Brimblecombe (2001: 24) raises the question as to whether we are witnessing a process of reinstitutionalization of psychiatry or an empowerment of other groups in the current climate. Reid (1989) is convinced that the medical hegemony continues, and Bracken and Thomas (1999a) remain concerned that the extension of psychiatric powers in the community will simply 'bring the institution into the community' (cited in Brimblecombe 2001: 24).

This brief overview of the history of madness, the creation of psychiatry and the treatment of people experiencing mental health problems has illustrated the evolution of psychiatry as a political as well as a medical process. However, the question remains: what is the psychiatric view on the nature of mental illness in the 21st century? Competing theories of mental illness will now be explored, illustrating a lack of agreement on the nature, causes and treatment of mental illness, and leading some to turn to narrative psychiatry and giving primacy to the voice of the user.

1.3 Theories of mental illness

It is asserted by Ingleby (1981: 23) that,

> The many conflicting viewpoints which flourish [in psychiatry] can be understood only in terms of the philosophical systems underlying them – prior beliefs about what people are, and how we should try to understand them – and that these philosophical systems are themselves based on moral or political priorities.

Although I will outline three theories of mental illness proffered by the psychiatric profession, Double (2005) has wisely stated that any view which criticizes or challenges the dominant medical model within psychiatry is now seen as 'anti-psychiatry'.

1.3.1 The medical model

Whilst undertaking my research in Bradford I had the opportunity to witness a 'ward round' at the local psychiatric hospital. It was a fascinating meeting, involving six professionals from the hospital, social services, the community resource centre and the new home treatment service. All eyes were on the psychiatrist for the ward, who was very much centre stage and seldom interrupted by his professional colleagues. Patients were brought in by the ward nurse one after the other and the psychiatrist usually asked a variation on the following three questions: 'are you sleeping okay?', 'are you eating okay?' and 'are you still taking the medication?' Based on the answers, the psychiatrist made an assessment of the patient's progress. Medication doses were altered, a different medication was prescribed, sometimes a course of ECT. An estimate was made of how long the patient would still need in hospital and the patient was then dismissed. Between seeing patients, a young social worker explained to the psychiatrist that one of her charges was currently on the ward. Her client had children and she was hoping the user could return home soon. The client had a diagnosis of 'manic depression'. The social worker asked the psychiatrist for some more information about the illness and what significance it would have in dealing with her client's problems. I noted down the conversation that followed:

Psychiatrist: 'Has she [the user] been taking the tablets?'
Ward Nurse: 'Yes, no outbursts…'

P: 'There is a pattern to it, when she gets out of control... she does suffer from psychosis... Briefly, it is a relapse of her psychosis, with regular medication it should settle down. How does she spend time on the ward?'

WN: 'On and off with the other clients – gets on well.'

P: 'It's a similar formula, it's psychosis, she relapses from time to time....'

Social Worker: 'Is it a long-term thing?'

P: 'Yes.'

SW: 'Maybe it can be controlled by medication?'

P: 'Yes, if she takes medication regularly and has regular support at home – both practical and emotional, both have an impact on her mental state – she should function reasonably well. She will need monitoring when she's taking medication.'

SW: 'She drinks, that might not help.'

P: 'Yes, that doesn't help but I'm not sure we can alter her lifestyle. Pills try to correct the chemical imbalance in the brain, alcohol will make it lob-sided, so it won't help. I refuse to treat patients who are still set on drinking.'

WN: 'She has nightmares where she says demons are coming out of the walls, and visual hallucinations.'

P: 'She sees or imagines?'

Community Psychiatric Nurse: 'Could try cognitive therapy.'

P: 'Personally, I don't think cognitive therapy is going to work. If a person is ill then they need treatment. Cognitive therapy will be a waste of money.'

This is a clear example of the medical model of psychiatry in action. The medical model (sometimes known as the 'biomedical model') states that mental illness is a disease of the brain. For example, it is the result of malfunctioning neurotransmitters that allow too much of one chemical or not enough of another chemical to the brain, thus causing irrational thought and/or behaviour. Given its ability to stabilize chemical imbalances in the brain, pharmacological medication is then the main treatment applied. Research is focused on brain neurology, identifying ever more precisely which mix of chemicals will work best with which mental illness. The medical model remains the dominant model within psychiatry. Double (2005), for example, notes that 'a recent statement from the American Psychiatric Association (APA) (2003) on the diagnosis and treatment of mental disorders maintained that schizophrenia and other mental disorders are serious neurobiological disorders'. In fact, the last decade of the 20th century saw a reasserting of this model, through an increase in neurological research and many new 'wonder drugs' in psychiatry. Putting this in an historical perspective the psychiatrists Bracken and Thomas (2001) comment,

> The Enlightenment promised that human suffering would yield to the advance of rationality and science. For its part, psychiatry sought to replace spiritual, moral, political, and folk understandings of madness with the technological framework of psychopathology and neuroscience. This culminated in the recent 'decade of the brain' and the assertion that madness is caused by neurological dysfunction, which can be cured by drugs targeted at specific neuroreceptors. It is now almost heretical to question this paradigm.

Nevertheless, serious questions continue to be raised about the legitimacy of the medical model both from within the profession and from outside. The concentration on mental illness as simply a brain illness denies human capacity for free thought independent of the physical hardware. The mind is reduced to the physical workings of our neuroreceptors. Over two centuries ago, this theory of mental illness was already causing the emerging profession sleepless nights, with John Haslam (1798) stating that '[t]he various and discordant opinions, which have prevailed in this department of knowledge, have led me to disentangle myself as quickly as possible from the perplexity of metaphysical mazes' (cited in Critical Psychiatry Network 2000). As we have seen in the development of psychiatry there has been a need for the justification of the profession as a legitimate part of medicine. The response had to be seen as scientific, with Moncrieff *et al.* (2005) confirming that 'the psychiatric profession has been inclined to favor biological models of mental disorder and physical treatments as a means of bolstering its credibility and claims to authority in the management of mental disorder'. Despite the claims of the dominant model of psychiatry, the ability to identify and treat mental illness in such an isolated way has been exaggerated. The inherent danger of a biological view of mental illness also leaves the profession open to claims of the pharmaceutical industry dictating psychiatric treatment (Moncrieff 2003). This increased medicalization of people's problems has reached epic proportions in the 21st century. Bracken and Thomas (1999c) explain,

> This biological trend is part of a wider cultural shift towards understanding ourselves in a technical idiom. All sorts of human

> difficulties are now regarded as the rightful concern of psychological experts and their knowledge. Scientific psychiatry and psychology tell us that human experience is 'something' which can be analyzed and explained in much the same way as other 'things' in the world. This is the key assumption of all technical and scientific approaches and underscores biological and cognitive developments. One of the great attractions of a technical paradigm is that it reveals a world which is open to prediction and manipulation. However, we should not forget that paradigms can conceal as much as they reveal. In their frantic efforts to convert the human world into something amenable to ever more manipulation and control, psychiatry and psychology obscure the essential mystery that lies at the heart of human experience.

The medical model has had its critics for many years. It ignores socio-economic factors, it ignores the power of psychiatry to label people as mental ill, it ignores its own political history and philosophical vocation and it ignores user explanations for illness. Two alternative views of mental illness will now be discussed. Despite the continued dominance of the medical model, these competing theories have left their mark on recent psychiatric thinking.

1.3.2 Interpretive psychiatry

The interpretative paradigm sees a crucial difference in human beings in their capacity for meaningful behaviour (or 'praxis') which cannot be either described or explained as if it were a 'thing'. Abandoning the positivism of the medical model, the distinction between describing and explaining ceases to be hard and fast 'since the two processes are combined in the single act of *interpretation*' (Ingleby 1981: 46, emphasis original). Interpretative psychiatry takes the form of 'normalizing' approaches to mental illness including the anti-psychiatry approach. Assumptions are made that *common sense* is capable of doing justice not only to ordinary behaviour but also to that of the mental patient. Scheff (1996), for example, argued that psychiatric illness was socially constructed just as physical ones were; the characteristics of 'mental illness' are prevalent in the 'normal' population, yet if a person is *labelled* 'sick' these states are overlooked. The popular form that interpretative psychiatry takes today can be summarized as the 'social model' (sometimes also as the 'psychosocial model' or even as the 'biopsychosocial model') of mental illness, which is keenly cited by many psychiatric professionals as relevant theory in explaining peoples decline into mental illness. This is summed up by

David Cooper (cited in Foucault 1967: viii), a leading figure in the 1960s anti-psychiatry movement, who stated,

> Recent psychiatric – or perhaps anti-psychiatric – research into the origins of the major form of madness in our age, schizophrenia, has moved round to the position that people do not in fact go mad, but are driven mad by others who are driven into the position of driving them mad by a peculiar convergence of social pressures.

Laing went further by claiming that there are simply different ways of interpreting and experiencing the world, and madness is just one of them. The anti-psychiatry movement rejected the scientific base of psychiatry and embraced different kinds of human experience. Similar to the ideas of recent therapists such as Rose (1999), what was seen by psychiatry as evidence of 'psychopathology' could in fact be different – even higher – states of being. Thus, Cooper (1967: 93) commented that 'psychotic experience may, with correct guidance, lead to a more advanced human state but only too often is converted by psychiatric interference into a state of arrest and stultification of the person'. It is worth noting that Cooper still uses the 'psychotic' label here and suggests the continued need for 'guidance' from the appropriate professionals.

Ingleby (1981) is also an advocate of the interpretative approach, though he believes in a more specific form known as 'depth hermeneutics', the chief example of which is psychoanalysis. In his opinion, the meanings of behaviour and experiences may not be consciously appreciated by either the agent or his fellows. The 'normalization' accounts leaves us questioning what is 'common sense' anyway? Ingelby argues that there needs to be a 'bridging' of the 'free will' and determinist approaches in psychiatry.

In bringing this debate more up-to-date, it is interesting that some of the strongest critics of psychiatry (for example, Breggin 1993; Masson 1989) have – like Ingleby – espoused the virtues of psychoanalysis, psychotherapy and other forms of psychological therapy (cognitive therapy is another current favourite, which brings together biomedical theory with the practice of psychology). Giving a different interpretation of events, Miller (1986) suggests this is less a case of changing paradigms than a more logical attempt to internally reform the dominant psychiatric ideology which is seen as too medical and somatic. These internal critiques come from two quarters;

> One of those is a modernizing group within psychiatry, or sometimes on its borders, that seeks to reform psychiatry by reducing the significance of the medical model and installing in its place a psychological model of disease and cure. The other is a more sociological mode of critique that equates medicalisation with social control, one that depicts psychology in a positive light, as something good and to be promoted against the evils of medicalisation.
>
> (1986: 24)

The former 'reformist' psychiatric response has offered a positive way forward for psychiatry and has allowed new approaches to seep into the profession without undermining its authority as the appropriate body to deal with mental disorders. Thus we can find such respected figures in psychiatry such as Anthony Clare questioning the categorization of 'schizophrenia' and calling for more flexibility in dealing with mental patients in the community (see Clare 1982). On the other hand, the latter approach is represented by commentators such as Pilgrim (1999), a clinical psychologist who presents regular critiques of psychiatric practice. He has argued that the 'treatability debate' surrounding the discussion of 'personality disorders' is 'based on a false premise of cure within the medical model of psychiatry', instead 'evidence-based intervention' should be considered (Pilgrim 1999: 7). Such has been the influence of interpretive psychiatry and the 'social model' of mental illness over the last 40 years that we now find esteemed psychiatrists such as Professor Sheila Hollins (2006) – President of the Royal College of Psychiatrists – strongly endorsing the 'importance of psychological therapies in the treatment of mental illness'.

1.3.3 Critical psychiatry

The third approach to mental illness from within psychiatry I broadly categorize as 'critical psychiatry'. This approach offers a similar critique of the medical model to that of interpretive psychiatry but also criticizes many psychological and psychotherapeutic treatments as well. They argue that treatment needs to be deconstructed and user-centred. The development of narrative approaches to psychiatry has come from these psychiatric theorists. As an example, Parker (1999) criticizes not only the practices of ECT and enforced medication within psychiatry but also some of the current practices of the British Psychological Association. One such practice is the 'psychologising [of] politics' through practices like psychotherapy (for example, Psychology Politics Resistance

1998), instead he would like to see more narrative and deconstructionist approaches to therapy (Parker 1999).

Similar ideas have also been promoted by other critical psychiatrists. In proposing the new term of 'post-psychiatry' for their work, Bracken and Thomas (1998: 17) argue that both the positivist and interpretive psychiatric theories have offered certain 'truths' about the nature of mental illness without challenging the internal logic of psychiatry itself, consequently psychiatry 'still promises the control of madness by reason, the conquest of disorder by rational technique'. We live in post-modern times, it is argued, and the promise of modernity now seems less attractive – the notion of any context-free 'truths' is in doubt. As a result,

> Psychiatry can no longer claim any privileged understanding of madness, alienation or distress. This is what we call post-psychiatry. However, the same applies to psychiatry's critics. Our argument is that those who adopt critical positions must abandon their own tendency to promise too much.
>
> (Bracken and Thomas 1998: 17)

The Critical Psychiatry Network (see www.critpsynet.freeuk.com), in which Parker, Bracken, Thomas and many other psychiatrists, critical therapists, counsellors and academics participate, offers an umbrella organization for professionals to discuss the power and politics of psychiatry and suggest new ways of working with people with mental health problems. Whilst user experience of distress and crises are real to them and should be treated as such, 'mental illness' and associated medical labels are no longer accepted as useful or valid. Instead, treatment must involve genuine dialogue with the user on an egalitarian basis. What has previously been seen by psychiatry as irrational behaviour and thought – thus, evidence of mental illness – should be accepted as having meaning and significance for users, and worked with on the basis of joint problem-solving.

I had the privilege to carry out research in Bradford with the psychiatrists Pat Bracken and Phil Thomas as participants, and this allowed me a unique opportunity to study the practical workings of these critical psychiatrists: would I witness an emergence of a genuinely new form of mental health care, where psychiatry is fractured and dispersed, with power passing to other groups and individuals? Or would I find a continuation of the medical model in the community? This will be investigated later in the book.

1.4 Psychiatry and medico-eclecticism

In 2001, Bracken and Thomas published a paper in the *British Medical Journal (BMJ)* calling on their colleagues to contemplate 'post-psychiatry' as a positive way forward for the profession. Using a critique of psychiatry's history and biomedical-focused treatment as the starting point, the consultants argued,

- faith in the ability of science and technology to resolve human and social problems is diminishing;
- this creates challenges for medicine, particularly traditional psychiatry;
- psychiatry must move beyond its 'modernist' framework to engage with recent government proposals and the growing power of service users;
- post-psychiatry emphasizes social and cultural contexts, places ethics before technology, and works to minimize medical control of coercive interventions;
- post-modernity provides doctors with an opportunity to redefine their roles and responsibilities.

The resulting 'rapid responses' to the paper – posted at the *BMJ*'s website – illustrates something quite significant about the current thinking about mental illness and treatment within psychiatry (many of the responses were from fellow consultants). There were those who chose to praise the article as 'enlightening' (Cuevas-Sosa 2001) and congratulate the authors for 'their courage in facing and naming the dehumanizing biological shibboleth of contemporary psychiatry' (Rapley 2001). Many more responses, however, were critical. As if to acknowledge Double's (2005) comment that any critic of the medical model is labelled as part of anti-psychiatry, a number of consultants denounced Bracken and Thomas as just that. According to Ranjith and Mohan (2001), for example, the authors' criticisms of psychiatry, 'are no more than recycled arguments of the antipsychiatry movement: their vision is high on ideals and low on practical utility'. Cabrera-Abreu and Milev (2001) went even further in their response entitled 'the sleep of reason produces monsters', claiming déjà vu in the criticisms of modern psychiatry and decrying the authors their 'pointless and vain attempt to reformulate psychiatry and mental illness under these [post-modern] conditions'. At the end of this rather pompous response, Cabrera-Abreu and Milev (2001) summed up the paper as attempting to aggravate, 'a pointless war between postmodernist psychiatrist [*sic*] and those who somewhat perplexed get along with the clinical work'.

Many of the other responses reflected Cabrera-Abreu and Milev's (2001) conclusion – many agreed there had been failures in psychiatry's past, but this did not mean there was a need for the total rejection of psychiatric practices in meeting the needs of people with mental health problems. Psychiatry must be pragmatic and clinical work had to be orientated to each individual's suffering. Too much theorizing and not enough practice makes psychiatry a dull boy. 'Rather than losing ourselves in a philosophical discussion, we prefer to see the faults and failings [of psychiatry] in a grossly under-resourced service', responded Melichar and Argyropoulos (2001), 'we prefer to leave our intellectual power struggles outside of the day-to-day care of the patients'. It is to this 'pragmatic psychiatry' that many of the responses belonged. 'Perhaps we are also practicing postpsychiatry' suggested Barron (2001), because their use of the 'bio-psycho-social model' in treating people with learning disabilities, 'has enabled us to begin to overcome the damaging split between medical and social models which dogged services for people with learning disabilities for so long'. Summating these points, Smith (2001) questioned whether Bracken and Thomas's arguments were radically new or simply 'an exercise in re-branding of the status quo of British psychiatry'. The author claimed that psychiatry in Britain had moved on from a primary focus on mental illness as a biological disorder to incorporate psychological and social models of distress in meeting the needs of mental health users. Smith (2001) concluded that he supported the authors' view:

> Psychiatrists who only work within a narrow biological framework can disadvantage and alienate some users of mental health services. However, I feel that their insights are hardly an earth-shattering revelation. The vast majority of psychiatrists of my acquaintance realise the need to understand 'social and cultural contexts', place 'ethics before technology' and work to 'minimise medical control of coercive interventions' [all citations from Bracken and Thomas's original article]. So is postpsychiatry that radical a departure from the way most psychiatrists practice in this country, or is it any departure at all?

The implications of the responses to Bracken and Thomas are clear: psychiatry is now eclectic in its approach to mental health problems and, thus, pragmatic in its treatment of users. There is a place for medical, psychological and social models in treatment options; none has primacy in reaching the needs of the individual. This version of the pragmatic progress of psychiatry, however, has been questioned by Colin Samson (1995a), who observed the treatment practices of consultant psychiatrists in the United Kingdom. In the face of changing mental health policy, Samson (1995a: 248) remarks that psychiatrists have developed the rhetoric of 'eclecticism' in their clinical practices though the fundamental orthodoxy of the biomedical viewpoint remains firmly intact. In his view,

> British psychiatry has been predominately biological in its aetiological theory, medical in its professional organization and political allegiance, and yet 'eclectic' in its self perception. That is, while biological medicine has provided the main source of knowledge for theory and practice, members of the profession have represented these enterprises as one engaging in wider domains within the social sciences. Although social theories of mental health have been forwarded, these have been present only on the margins of the profession.

From his research on consultants in Bristol, Samson found that non-medical approaches are considered and used if available (for example, massage, acupuncture, aromatherapy), but they are not the dominant treatment model and can often be discarded in favour of biomedical solutions. The point made here is that the psychiatric profession sees itself as progressing and adapting new approaches to its work, whilst the status quo remains unchallenged and unchanged on the whole. Concluding this point, Samson (1995a: 251) comments,

> The adoption of an eclectic belief system may be seen as contributing to the maintenance of medical dominance. The presentation of eclecticism connotes a particular authority, an intellectual and therapeutic flexibility which enables the psychiatrist to handle the wide range of mental conditions encountered by the mental health services.

This can be seen as one attempt by a professional group to maintain their dominance in the marketplace. Turner (1987: 155) explains that the professional dominance of certain occupational groups is 'clearly grounded in the possession of a body of knowledge which is a crucial feature of the exercise of professional power'. In maintaining medical dominance, argues Turner, it is necessary to preserve and extend access to its clientele whilst at the same time limiting and subordinating professionals in related areas. Thus, internally, the psychiatric profession sees itself as having a broader range of skills than other professional workers in the mental health field, given their ability to treat both the body and mind as well as relating to patients in psychological, social and medical terms. This accomplishment, however, has only succeeded as far as seeing the mind as biological matter (Capra 1982; Samson 1995a; Turner 1987, 1995).

Although not unheard of within public psychiatry, alternative approaches to mental health tend to come from outside the statutory sector. These approaches draw on a range of philosophies including humanistic psychology, psychoanalysis, spiritualism, the New Age movement and user empowerment. The overwhelming difference between these 'holistic' approaches and public psychiatry is that 'the alternative eclecticism is not aligned to a privileging of medical knowledge' (Samson 1995a: 258). Consequently, within the alternative provision there is more emphasis placed on counselling, psychotherapy, practical help and therapeutic communities. Above all, there is a belief in the social aetiology of mental illness.

1.5 Conclusion

This chapter has detailed the rise of psychiatry and the development of theories of mental illness. In the 21st century, the debate about what mental illness actually is continues. Inwardly, psychiatry perceives itself as a progressive profession within medicine; eclectic in approach and pragmatic in treatment. Yet there is a continued belief in the medical model and reliance on pharmaceutical treatment, despite an overestimation of the benefits of such treatment. Psychiatry has become a powerful political force with the unique skills to treat the mentally disturbed. They have strong professional associations protecting their interests, such as the APA, and multinational pharmaceutical firms ready to pay the bills (for the latest example of the dire consequences of such 'partnerships' see BBC 2007, which highlights the relationship between the pharmaceutical company GlaxoSmithKline and the respected psychiatrist Martin Keller in selling the drug Paroxetine, despite its links to suicide in teenagers; for a more general survey of the invention of new diseases by drug companies see Moynihan and Cassels 2005). Despite the big question mark that hangs above psychiatric beliefs about mental illness, the voices of detractors are confined to the margins and to people outside of the profession. These voices include, of course, the mental health users themselves.

Since the late 1950s, the psychiatric paternalistic public sphere has been challenged, firstly by civil rights groups and then by the radical anti-psychiatry movement which saw the birth of the user movement in the late 1960s. Critical campaigning groups – such as MIND in the United Kingdom – created an oppositional public sphere to psychiatry and introduced user voices into the mental health debate (see Crossley 1997). With decarceration and community care there has been specific provision laid out for the involvement of the 'consumer' in planning, provision and treatment (see Perring 1992). It has therefore been argued that there is a need for a 'radical shift in [mental health worker] views on the relationship between service providers, service users, and among the different groups of providers' (Perring 1992: 170). Beumont (1992: 544) argues that this calls for a 'need to understand patients' experiences' of their illness. The neglect of such approaches by psychiatry for much of the 20th century, 'may be to the detriment of patient welfare' (Beumont 1992: 544).

With psychiatry taking a more overt interest in phenomenological approaches – which in turn express a 'user-friendly' system of operation – it can be seen to be offering alternatives. With the rise of welfare management, mental health administrators have been keen to evaluate service delivery and consumer views, and the results often reflect badly on psychiatry and what is often seen as the process of 'depersonalised' service (see Peloquin 1993). As a result, commentators such as Mattingly (1991) have called on psychiatry to develop the more rounded approaches of phenomenology, which have been 'neglected as an articulating and legitimising framework for practice' (cited in Peloquin 1993: 831). Further to this, it is argued that user narratives need to be taken seriously by psychiatry. Users have commented 'that practitioners act in a way that belies any client of understanding', yet due to the special connection made with practitioners through the illness process, 'practitioners become significant others but do not seem to recognise their heightened significance' (Peloquin 1993: 831).

The burgeoning consumer groups in mental health are calling, amongst other things, for a 'new partnership' between doctors and patients, psychiatrists and users, which has greater humanism, allows the user a greater say in treatment and gives credibility to user experiences as relevant and legitimate. As the hierarchical structure of the therapist–client relationship can indirectly reinforce feelings of inadequacy and powerlessness, Miller (1994) has noted that a narrative approach can facilitate a more equal relationship with the therapist. In Chapter 2 the move towards narratives and the contemplation of user life stories will be discussed.

2
Narratives

> The psychiatrist had seemed to be the typical psychiatrist, he seemed extremely eccentric. We seemed to talk for hours about nothing in particular and yet he seemed to be able to work out what I was thinking about, so there was obviously method in his madness as it were.
>
> (Simon)

2.1 Summary

Chapter 1 looked in some detail at the rise of the psychiatric profession, the changing institutional status, changes in treatment models and competing theories of mental illness. It was noted that modern psychiatry sees itself as eclectic and pragmatic, whilst the reality is a continued reliance on the medical model and pharmaceutical medication as the main treatment option. Nevertheless, this chapter will show that there has been increasing interest in 'the narrative approach' to treatment with mental health users. Likewise, the humanities are also turning towards narratives as a more valid way of understanding people's lives than 'traditional' methods of research. Post-modernist theory and writings have been influential here and some time is devoted to investigating the main arguments. Towards the end of the chapter, a compromise definition and method for carrying out narrative research is given. This 'narrative method' will be demonstrated later in the book through work with mental health users in Bradford.

2.2 Background

Stories are a fundamental way for humans to communicate and understand one another. 'When people converse, write, sing, chat on the phone and e-mail', note Lapsley *et al.* (2002: 3), 'they often tell stories about themselves and the people they know'. Despite the possibility of exaggeration or distortion within such communication, these stories impose an order and meaning on our lives. Such stories have been imparted throughout human existence, with some famous early examples being cave paintings, aboriginal stone markings and Egyptian hieroglyphics (Thompson 1978). Since the Enlightenment and the dawning of the Age of Reason, however, human stories have been confined to the arts where fictional works can be seen in contrast to the world of science. The modernist project of science has attempted to objectify the world. It has been assumed that laws for human behaviour can be uncovered in the same way as laws for innate objects.

In the last few decades this modernist worldview has been questioned. There has been a turn towards cultural anthropology, literary theory and post-modern philosophy. As a result, there has been a coming together of historians, social scientists and the humanities with increased intellectual collaboration taking place. Narrative has been one emerging point of interaction between them. Nash (1990: xi) has seen these developments as part of an attempt by modern culture to begin 'speaking with itself':

> Whole movements have sprung up (within ethnomethodology, psycho-linguistics, social constructionism, critical legal studies), groups in the physical sciences, the social sciences, the professions, seeking to apply techniques first largely evolved in literary and linguistic studies to the scrutiny of their own patterns of communication, conception and perception.

Within the same time period, the ideas of 'post-modern' writers have increased in influence for many in the human sciences. The post-modern critiques of Western science and their focus on language play a crucial role in the current study of psychiatric user narratives, so some time is spent here surveying some of the main arguments as well as the impact on social constructionist study which has been informed by such writers.

2.3 Post-modernism

Lyotard has argued that the world is currently in a 'post-modern' condition following the transformations at the end of the 19th century. These changes altered the 'rules' within the sciences, literature and the arts. 'The society of the future', argues Lyotard (1979: xxiv),

> Falls less within the province of a Newtonian anthropology (such as structuralism or systems theory) than a pragmatics of language particles. There are many different language games – a heterogeneity of elements. They only give rise to institutions in patches – local determinism.

Post-modernist writers argued that science also has a narrative which appears as a set of 'rules' by which it operates and organizes in the same way as other disciplines do. It relies especially in the 21st century on language and linguistics discourse to legitimize its actions. As Lyotard states of science, 'it is obliged to legitimate the rules of its own game. It then produces a discourse of legitimisation with respect to its own status, a discourse called philosophy' (1979: xxii). Derrida also alludes to this point when he says, 'my central question is: how can philosophy as such appear to itself as other than itself, so that it can interrogate and reflect upon itself in an original manner?' (cited in Norris 1987: 26).

This deconstructionist approach has criticized Western science for the creation of a powerful system of knowledge that holds an illusion of seeking 'truth' and discovering 'facts' about the world, whilst being culturally and historically specific. It is argued that science is a system of belief akin to religion in which shared cultural meaning, through a shared language, has constructed the idea of a 'reality' that we can have knowledge of. As Norris (1987: 65) asserts of language,

> Spoken words are the signs we adopt to communicate thoughts and ideas. Written words are the secondary symbols that stand in for speech and so at one further remove assist in the process of communication. Already there is the outline of a hierarchy here, a descending order of priority in which writing ranks a very poor third on account of its irrevocable distance from origin, truth and self-present meaning.

Similarly, Wittgenstein has questioned the possibility of a 'purely logical language' by which we can make sense of our world as science claims to. 'It is a strange paradox', wrote Wittgenstein, 'that what would appear to be the most common, public and accessible world, the world of immediate experience, should be the most private, isolated and inaccessible' (cited in Finch 1995: 22). So, in place of modern philosophy's question 'what does it mean to think?' (as originally formulated by Descartes), Foucault asks 'what does it mean to speak?'

The concepts of 'scientific thought' and 'rationality' are important parts of modern Western culture, though they actually tell us more about our own construction of a social world than about an actual world which science can investigate. Canguilhem (1994: 76) explains Foucault's idea as follows:

> A culture is a code that orders human experiences in three respects – linguistic, perceptual, practical; a science or a philosophy is a theory or an interpretation of that ordering. But the theories and interpretations in question do not apply directly to human experience. Science and philosophy presupposes the existence of a network or configuration of forms through which cultural productions are perceived. These forms already constitute, with respect to that culture, knowledge different from the knowledge constituted by sciences and philosophies. This network is invariant and unique to a given epoch, and thus identifiable through references to it.

Foucault gives an example for this theory of cultural relativity: we might believe from a rationalist perspective of history that the 17th century saw the passing of the old beliefs in superstition and magic to make way for the entry of nature and scientific order. But, he explains, 'what we must grasp and attempt to reconstitute are the modifications that affected knowledge itself, at that archaic level which makes possible both knowledge itself and the mode of being of what is to be known' (cited in Canguilhem 1994: 76).

For Foucault it is the study of language and the power of knowledge through use of language which should be the basis of study, not what has been defined by a given epoch as the way things are. Canguilhem notes that language, since the Renaissance, has become the instrument for manipulation by philosophers and scientists. Language is no longer simply the signature or mark of things, but an 'organ allowing them to be composed in a universal tableau of identities and differences; a means not for revealing order, but for dispensing it' (1994: 77).

Through their discrediting of the 'grand narratives' of science, Botting (1995: 88) argues that thinkers such as Foucault and Lyotard have turned history into a series of stories involving a host of language games. The result is that society becomes a fluid entity where we can be certain of nothing:

> This general explosion and implosion of images, signs and meanings caused by new technologies and post-modern practices leads to history's decomposition into stories and the subject's dissolution: they become plural and decentred selves, their reality virtually absorbed into the image machine of technical reproduction where cultures proliferate and consume themselves.

The post-modern paradigm and social construction of reality has begun to influence many different disciplines within the social sciences, the basic premise being that reality is not hard and fast but is constructed, usually in dialogue with other people (Anderson and Goolishian 1992; Gergen and Kaye 1992; Horner 1995; Saari 1991; Stern 1985). One aspect of the new paradigm is the focus on language and storytelling as the creation of individuals' beliefs about their lives. Horner (1995: 10–11) remarks that such theorists have, 'raised to the level of constant dialogue in the field of psychiatry, psychology, and social work the idea of narrative as formative and, therefore, potentially trans-formative', the assumption being that we can fundamentally 're-author' our lives through the stories we tell. Thus, narratives for post-structural theorists are central to the understanding of human beings. Indeed, they are one of the few avenues left to explore which might enlighten social theorists about the world. It is because of this focus on language, linguistics and the human narrative by post-structuralists that they are the major theorists to examine narratives and narrative theory in depth. The influence of such writings, together with the disillusionment with the medical model and the restricted modes of treatment in current practice, has seen a recent move within psychiatry to explore user narratives. These developments will now be discussed.

2.4 The psychiatric narrative

More literature on narrative approaches to psychiatry and related fields has appeared during the 1990s and 2000s, signalling that the profession is taking user narratives much more seriously than ever before. In this section, I discuss the psychiatric discourse on user narratives and whether this signifies 'radical change' in the focus of psychiatry as some have argued (for example, Horner 1995) or the continued self-perception of 'eclecticism' which justifies psychiatry's continued autonomy in biomedical matters (e.g. Samson 1995a).

One of the most comprehensive works on the possibilities of psychiatry taking a narrative approach to illness has been Arthur Kleinman's

(1988) book *The Illness Narratives*. As a psychiatrist himself, Kleinman argues extensively for the centrality of a person's life experiences in understanding their worldview and the meanings of their illness. He comments that the interpretation of illness meanings and the complexities of personal relationships should not be seen by the profession as peripheral tasks, 'they constitute, rather, the point of medicine. These are the activities with which the practitioner should be engaged. The failure to address these issues is a fundamental flaw in the work of doctoring' (Kleinman 1988: 253).

Kleinman's argument concurs with a number of studies from psychiatry and social psychology. In their study of user accounts of mental illness, Estroff *et al.* (1992) illustrated the interdependence of accounts of and for illness and self. Individual meanings were given for users' illnesses and these appeared to be more important than formal psychiatric diagnoses and treatment. The research suggested that *individual understanding* of the problem – rather than formal psychiatric diagnoses and other medical factors – had a strong influence on the view of self. Palombo (1992) noted serious clinical problems in current psychoanalytic paradigms and reliance on inconsistencies in professional assumptions which inform clinical theory. He proposed a new conceptualization of mental health problems based on the development and organization of meanings in self-narratives. There was a need for practising clinicians to place more emphasis on the personal meanings of human conduct and less on factual, objective methods of analysing behaviour, otherwise one was likely to misread motives that lie behind behaviour. Further to this, Lee and Dwyer (1995) suggested psychiatry should go beyond simply providing care for users, to look at systems of relations through 'co-constructed narratives' from the patient and family, the professionals, the health care teams and others to be able to understand and explain the relation between physical, psychological, social and vocational aspects of the user.

In attempting to define what the 'illness narrative' is and how it can be explored by psychiatry, Kleinman (1988) outlines a number of cases of chronic illness he has dealt with in the past, illustrating the impossibility of separating the 'diseased' body from the self and the wider social world. There are necessary interconnections between physiological processes, meanings and relationships.

> The study of the process by which meaning is created in illness brings us into the everyday reality of individuals like ourselves, who must

> deal with the exigent life circumstances created by suffering, disability, difficult loss, and threat of death.
>
> (1988: xiii)

The illness narrative tells us about how life problems are created, controlled and made meaningful. They are shaped by our cultural values and social relations, and will affect our self-perception of illness and health as well as the way we monitor our body and act towards bodily symptoms and complaints. Fundamentally, Kleinman reiterates that *illness has meaning* for a person and to understand the personal narrative is to understand something fundamental about illness, care and perhaps life generally. In his opinion, the medical system has unfortunately done, 'just about everything to drive the practitioners' attention away from the experience of illness' (1988: xiv), contributing to the alienation of the chronically ill person from their practitioner. Kleinman clearly aligns the reason for this with the dominance of the biomedical model in psychiatry and the secularized practice of separating the body from the mind. Looking at non-Western cultures, he notes a more integrated view of the person as an organic part of a sociocentric world – 'a communication system involving exchanges with others' (1988: 11; see also Kleinman 1986).

Citing a number of his own clinical cases, Kleinman demonstrates how patients – who would normally have been labelled as suffering from severe mental illnesses – were in fact in deep distress due to life factors and historical events which surrounded their health problems (for example, a woman with diabetes who had had her foot amputated and was distressed about her ability to cope with the further pain and suffering of her illness; a young man who was suffering from leg pains and had difficulty communicating with his father). It would appear that Kleinman extracted long accounts of life circumstances and patients' feelings towards their illness over many sessions (sometimes lasting for years). And *interpretation* would seem to be the key to understanding the illness narrative of patients and, thus, their explanations of distress and trauma.

This 'narrative approach' in psychiatry should not be confused with the psychoanalysis of patients. The problem with psychoanalytic interpretations of illness, according to Kleinman, is that such practitioners are dissatisfied with the 'surface' level analysis and 'reach for "deeper" meanings for which there is usually little clinical or scientific justification. A single-minded quest for psychoanalytic reality can dehumanize the patient every bit as much as the numbing reductionism of an obsessively biomedical investigation' (1988: 42).

So, unlike psychoanalysis, the doctor–patient relationship which utilizes an illness narrative approach is a call for a surface-level interpretation, explanation and shared meaning of a given life story. As Eisenberg (1981: 245) has stated,

> The decision to seek medical consultation is a request for interpretation.... Patient and doctor together reconstruct the meaning of events in a shared mythopoesis.... Once things fall into place; once experience and interpretation appear to coincide; once the patient has a coherent 'explanation' which leaves him no longer feeling the victim of the inexplicable and the uncontrollable, the symptoms are, usually, exorcised.

How new is this focus on user narratives? Horner (1995: 11) reminds us that Freud and the various psychoanalytic schools that followed him certainly believed in narrative: 'clients were encouraged to tell stories, sometimes long ones and sometimes merely snippets, while he [Freud] listened with evenly suspended or hovering attention and occasionally made interpretations' (1995: 11). Although these narrative stories were seen as important, Horner remarks that the therapist's search for the historical truth (or seminal event) was the key to analysing and understanding the particular pathology. Many psychiatrists have, similarly, paid attention to user histories to understand better the background to a mental crisis (see also Korchin 1976; Stevens 1976; Sundberg *et al.* 1983).

It has been argued, however, that such linear causality is being questioned by several paradigm shifts in mental health (Horner 1995). Firstly, there has been a questioning of historical truths and of scientific methods. Secondly, a questioning of the possibility of a single casual relationship to be found for 'mental illness' and 'psychopathology'. With the aid of phenomenological philosophies in psychiatry (see Beumont 1992) it has been highlighted that there are numerous accounts and interpretations of experience, and that the psychiatrist is no less immune to value judgements than the user. Spence (1982) therefore believes we should think in terms of 'constructions' rather than 'reconstructions' of the past, with historical material treated as a 'creation' rather than the truth of what happened 'back then' (cited in Horner 1995: 11–12). The effect is most pronounced in social constructionist theories of dialogue and narrative. Gergen and Kaye (1992) state that psychiatrists have stories to tell as well as the patients – implicit in the professional narrative is a number of beliefs such as that there is a cause for mental illness; that the cause of this illness can be located within the client; that there are diagnoses for mental illness; and that there is a means for eradicating or containing the mental illness (see Horner 1995: 12). As Gergen (1994: 242) remarks of these therapist narratives,

> Significant questions must be raised about the traditional practice of replacing the client's stories with the fixed and narrow alternatives of the modern therapist. There is no justification outside the small community of like-minded therapists for hammering the client's complex and richly detailed life into a single, preformulated narrative, a narrative that may be of little relevance or promise for the client's subsequent life conditions.

The logic of psychiatry's narrative denies the legitimacy of the user narrative. Some have argued that this is necessary as mental health users have 'a true dysfunction in narrative production', and that psychiatry 'corrects' this cognitive functioning as the user gains insight through treatment (see Chaika and Lambe 1989: 407). This view has been challenged by a number of studies which suggest that, in certain subtle ways, a psychiatric narrative is *imposed* (rather than *negotiated* through treatment) upon the user through the auspices of neutral medical practices such as written and oral medical procedures. Charon (1992: 116), for example, has commented that 'a close reading of the written and oral transactions of medicine rewards the critic with a textual anatomy of belief, power, and ontological fears in which the words themselves carry weight'.

In studying 'writing as performance', Barrett (1988: 265) looked at psychiatric writings and how they might affect the identities of patients and their perceptions of their illness. One crucial transformation that was noted was the move from descriptions such as 'person suffering from schizophrenia' to 'schizophrenic': a move from a temporary habitus to an embodied 'ill' self, a move from temporary to permanent illness. The writing processes carried out by psychiatric staff in the presence of users was also heavily weighted to the user's entrance into the system. As Barrett points out,

> Although writing was crucial during the induction of a patient into a career of mental illness, there was no corresponding writing process

> through which the patient was transformed back into health. *The concept of officially writing a patient out of schizophrenia into health was foreign to psychiatric staff,* who characteristically reacted with some amusement among themselves when patients made a request for a written 'statement of mental health'.
>
> (1988: 292–3, emphasis added)

So engagement with the psychiatric system can often lead to a distinct labelling process through emphasizing users as 'ill' rather than in a state of 'wellness', in turn causing all the real effects that this process can entail. Charon (1992: 115) reiterates, 'to write "this unfortunate 72-year-old woman" at the head of a consult note sentences the patient to a slow but certain death'. Such a dominant medical aetiology is also transferred through dialogue and conversational exchange with the user, as Oliver Sacks admits, 'there's a part of me that almost *has* to organise clinical perception into a narrative, as well as theoretically.... *Subsequently, I think, the patient comes to share the story, and the story gets modified*' (cited in Showalter 1992: 24, first emphasis original, second emphasis added).

Showalter, who has studied the construction of the 'hysterical narrative' by medicine, agrees with Sack's statement, concluding that 'doctors stories [tend] to dominate medical discourse, while patients stories [are] modified' (1992: 24). Whilst the user narratives may be fluid and multifaceted, they are 'dumbed-down' by a biomedical model which seeks some ordering of experience through generalizability and categorization of each 'disorder' encountered. In this way user stories are disempowered by contact with mental health professionals. Kirmayer (1992: 339) believes this is down to the psychiatrist's inability to understand the metaphorical nature of user narratives, commenting,

> Part of what makes the patient's self-description unintelligible to the biomedical physician is the practitioner's tendency to take the metaphorical constructions of illness experience for literal statements within the empirical realm of biomedicine. Language is treated not as a personal expression but as a transparent universal code. But 'blood' for the patient is not 'blood' for the physician. The inability to see the metaphoric and contextual basis of discourse limits the physician's comprehension of the patient's life world.

This problem is illustrated by Saris' (1995) account of a life history of a user labelled as 'schizophrenic'. It was found that 'the subject at once acknowledges his (occasionally) profoundly altered phenomenological sense of himself and his surroundings, while struggling against his engulfment by a body of knowledge, psychiatry, which, in his eyes, sees little of him beyond an illness label' (1995: 39).

The implication from a number of critics inside the psy-complex (e.g. Parker 1999) is that the reductionism of the biomedical model in psychiatry (or the following of a 'caseness approach', as described by Susko 1994) is damaging to the user and should be replaced by the more 'humane' 'narrative approach'. The aforementioned research on the medical oral and writing traditions, however, suggest that the power differentials between professional and patient across the various fields are maintained despite the introduction of such approaches. Masson (1989) is one of the few who has suggested that the abuse of power can be carried through into therapeutic approaches beyond psychiatry, whether in counselling sessions, in psychotherapy or through other alternatives to psychiatry. The area of therapy remains grey on the subject of power, though social constructionist therapists have raised the question themselves: 'if the concept of care is sacrificed, the function of therapy is also placed in question. If there are no problems in reality and no solutions, then how is therapy justified?' (Gergen 1994: 244). Like Parker (1999), there is talk of being 'sensitive' to one's narrative, 'empowering' the user narrative and reaching 'joint solutions' in the meeting of therapist and user narratives. There is a suggestion that success in taking this narrative approach to therapy depends on the therapist's ability to change the interaction with the user. It is therefore implied that the therapist is the one with the power to change and to set the therapeutic agenda. In this way it is difficult to see how this psy-route is anymore productive for the user than being part of mainstream psychiatry.

Despite these problems of the turn to narrative within psychiatry, it is still useful to survey the proposed methods for extracting user narratives. How does one proceed in researching the points of local determinism and what can we make of the resulting texts? This is answered in the following sections with reference to social constructionists, personality theorists and social scientists that have developed lines of narrative study. It will become clear that both the definition and the application of the 'narrative approach' remain contentious.

2.5 Social constructionism

One of the main social constructionist thinkers to study narratives in depth, Gergen (1994) proposes a relational view of self-conception. That is, a view of the self as a narrative given meaning through ongoing relationships in the public sphere, rather than based on private cognitive processes of the individual (for example, self-conception, schemas, self-esteem). Singer (1995: 256) notes that 'personality psychologists are prone to look more at an individual's efforts to find unity across narratives, rather than to emphasize the multiplicity of narrative generated by a post-modern culture'. The social constructionists challenge this traditional notion of a core identity by which we can measure a person's actions.

According to Gergen (1994: 186), we use the self-narrative or story to 'identify ourselves to others and to ourselves'. But unlike some other accounts of narrative, Gergen does not see narratives as a possession of an individual but rather the product of social interchange. 'In effect', says Gergen, 'to be a self with a past and potential future is not to be an independent agent, unique and autonomous, but to be immersed in interdependency' (1994: 186). This view of the self links one's actions and subsequent events to past actions and experiences; indeed, this is seen as the only way that actions and experiences represented through self-narratives can be understood and placed in context.

Gergen defines 'self-narratives' as 'an individual's account of the relationships among self-relevant events across time' (1994: 187). It is argued that a person's present identity comes about as the result of a collected life story. Yet Gergen is keen to separate these social constructionist ideas from the work of colleagues in other branches of psychology (for example, cognitive psychologists, rule-role theorists, constructivists, phenomenologists, existentialists and personalogists). Some psychologists place an emphasis on the individual whereas Gergen and other social constructionists see self-narratives as 'forms of social accounting or public discourse' (1994: 188). From this point of view the identification of the self is very much formed and interpreted through social action and social interpretation. The self-narrative becomes a way of translating and making sense of a person's life to others.

Though not endorsing cultural determinism, Gergen believes that it is only through interacting with other people that narrative skills are acquired, rather than an individual being acted upon by others. So although social constructionists contest the existence of a social reality external to the self, they also contest the idea of the isolated individual who can create narrative without recourse to interaction with others. The social constructionists do not study self-narratives to find 'the truth' about the world, rather they aim to understand through narratives the process by which a sense of 'what is true' is created by people. Gergen takes this further by stating that it is largely due to existing narrative forms that 'telling the truth' has become an intelligible act.

Narratives for social constructionists are not simply a way of telling someone (or oneself) about one's life, but are actually seen as a means by which a person constructs their identity. The self is in a state of flux and there is no one story. People can constantly change their life narrative and thus their self-conception. It is also believed that the narrative which informs identity will tend to invite certain actions whilst discouraging others. Narratives will tend to accentuate periods of particular significance whether positive or negative to a person: it may be the 'long struggle upwards' or the 'gradual decline' in one's narrative, rather than accentuating a life which goes round and round and would appear to be of no particular consequence.

Social constructionists therefore investigate these points of self-perceived 'highs' and 'lows' in the study of narratives. For example, Gergen and Gergen (1988) asked adolescents about events which occurred at the most positive and negative points of their life. The writers have also studied the life experiences of old people, asking them about their happiest days, and exploring why they had changed and in what direction. Gergen emphasizes the subjectivity of narratives; they 'are not the products of life itself, they are constructions of life' (1994: 201). But far from being by-products of life, from this point of view self-conceptions are driven largely from available narrative conventions. Social constructionist theories have heightened the awareness of the use of narrative as a way of re-evaluating approaches to the study of the individual. If we take Horner as a relevant example, it is argued that social constructionist theories of narrative should be taken seriously by psychoanalysts in their therapy sessions with clients. Horner (1995: 13–14, emphases original) comments, 'if we begin to now believe, as the post-modernists do, that knowledge, too, is socially constructed, then one story is no better than another. The therapist's story is just *another* one, rather than a *definite* one'. Horner concludes that therapists should recognize their own subjectivities, be open with the client, be more personal with them, create space for dialogue and try to get away from the 'tilted relationship' towards a more equal one. Palombo (1992: 259), for example, suggests that extracting narratives from children allows for the expression of unique interpretations of particular life episodes:

> The interpretations given to events by the child are woven into a historical account that has coherence, and that ultimately becomes his or her life narrative. Such narratives play a powerful role during a

person's life, and continue to be reshaped by experience during the life cycle.

2.6 Personality theorists

Although social constructionism has had a degree of impact on personality theorists (for example, psychologists, psychoanalysts, psychiatrists and other groups of therapists), most of the latter remain within a structuralist outlook. There is still a strong belief in the possibility of uncovering 'true' and accurate explanations for human behaviour. The emphasis remains on the core identity and individual traits of a person. These personality theorists have not questioned this fundamental premise as Gergen and others have. Rather, a shift in focus by these theorists has come about due to the possibilities of studying personal narratives, which might tell us something more fundamental about human behaviour than by utilizing more 'scientific methods' of investigation. This general disillusionment with what has been seen as the more 'rigorous' methods of collecting data on individuals has been noted by Baumeister and Newman (1994: 676) who comment that 'in recent years a growing body of research has noted that much of the thinking of ordinary people does not follow the patterns of inference, altercation, and generalisation that science itself favours'.

Mattingly and Garro (1994) outline a heightened interest in narratives in many fields of enquiry, including medicine, with a preoccupation for narrative as a mode of thought. Narrative modes of thought are seen as being grounded in particular human actions for these theorists. The study of narratives is possibly our most fundamental way of understanding our lives in time:

> Through narratives we try to make sense of how things have come to pass and how our actions and the actions of others have helped shape our history; we try to understand who we are becoming by reference to where we have been.
>
> (Mattingly and Garro 1994: 771)

However, Baumeister and Newman (1994: 676) believe that there are specific *reasons* why self-narratives give sense to experience. These are, a need for people to interpret experiences relative to purposes, 'which may be either objective goods or subjective fulfilment states'; a need to seek value and justification by constructing stories that define actions and intentions as right and good; a need to seek a sense of efficacy by making stories that contain information about how to exert control; or a need to seek a sense of self-worth by creating stories that portray themselves as attractive and competent. 'With this framework', argue Baumeister and Newman, 'narratives are effective means of making sense of experience' (1994: 676). The authors suggest that studying narratives can be a vital first step towards the understanding of an event. They also imply that from such understanding, inferences and deductions towards generalizations or causal theories can be made. They conclude that 'understanding the construction of narrative should...be one goal of social cognition' (1994: 688).

Baumeister and Newman further describe the work of Bruner (1986) and Zukier (1986), who distinguished between two different ways of structuring and processing information – the 'paradigmatic' and the 'narrative' modes of thought. The paradigmatic mode of thought, 'transcends the particular in favour of abstraction' (1994: 677). Moral rules and inferences of the person involve paradigmatic thinking 'insofar as they consist in setting up generalisations that subsume the individual events'. In contrast, narrative modes of thought are context-sensitive and temporarily structured, giving coherence to stories about particular experiences. As Baumeister and Newman put it, 'narrative is the mode of thought that best captures the experiential particularity of human action and intentionally, and it involves reasons, intentions, beliefs and goals' (1994: 677).

Towards the extreme empiricist end of these theorists are Abell (1987) and others (for example, Abbott 1993; Fararo 1993; Michaelson-Kanfer 1993) who in studying narratives set out 'to provide a rigorous framework in which the formulation of rules...for the analysis of connected sequences of human actions can be accomplished' (Abell 1987: 1). For Abell (1993: 94) narratives are the 'structure of interconnected, socially situated actions (and forbearances) [which] account for (or explain) the generation of specific outcomes'. Abell's definition is quantitatively based, concerned as it is with the relationship between an individual's narrative, their actions and the outcomes of those actions. He is not concerned with the problem of interpretation of the narrative or the context of the story itself, but with the formation of mathematical theory which will account successfully for action and the possible generalizability of human interaction with reference to narrative analysis. For example, Abell comments that 'social scientists should write stories accounting for the occurrence of a given event and then go on to ask how generalizable the story is, in generating similar or identical events' (1984: 309). The generalizability of the event (the action or interaction) is of key importance here.

Abell is concerned to outline these sequences as they lend themselves to the further analysis of 'social reality'. Taking a deterministic view, he believes that 'things come about in the social world because people in context (to include their previously acquired values and beliefs) bring them about by their actions' (Abell 1987: 1). Abell acknowledges that narratives not only describe actions but also explain what is happening in the social world, but believes that the 'natural language' found in narratives can be translated into a 'computer-readable' form which will 'eventually render qualitative analysis as routine as the statistical procedures now available to the variable-centered method' (Abell 1987: 2). This idea puts Abell and his colleagues at odds with other theorists who have argued that narratives are an interpretation, a version or a construction of 'reality', but not a direct 'truth' about an objective social world. It is also in contrast to the anti-empiricist stand of most other narrative theorists. Generally, Abell's approach is not flexible enough to the possibility of variance within narratives produced through different contexts. Issues of place, time, culture, language and understanding within the production of narratives are ignored in favour of a fixed notion of narrative rule formulation. Language is seen as a neutral – rather than a politically and culturally manipulated – process by such theorists.

2.7 Social science

Like Abell, some social scientists do agree that it is possible to quantify narratives. Heath (1986: 84), for example, suggests that 'at the broadest level, narratives are verbalised memories of past or ongoing experiences'. Looking at cross-cultural narratives, she remarks that all societies can recognize and produce narratives in 'predictable, coherent organised patterns of structure and content' (1986: 85), but may produce the narratives in different ways, whether in oral or written forms. Likewise, Taylor *et al.* (1986: 197) define 'personal narratives' as 'accounts of significant events that participants provide about themselves for the attention of interested parties'. It is argued by these writers that whereas personal narratives were once one of the main sources of information for clinical or social psychologists, they are now a method with some objective, quantifiable and reliable status for social scientists. The narrative can be either spoken or written, and in written form may allow us to discover 'previously hidden aspects of the patient's world' (Goldberg 1973, cited in Taylor *et al.* 1986).

Within other branches of social science a similar view is taken for defining and studying narrative. Personal discourse becomes a way to reflect on wider structural issues – it allows more individual insight and understanding of actions, motivations and cognitions which are often overlooked as a significant variable in the shaping of different social systems across time and culture. This is illustrated by Hart (1992) who believes that the narrative has a 'dual role' for historians. Firstly, it is a means of representing life in a given culture and, secondly, narratives allow historians to study the crucial dynamics of historical change as perceived by people at the time. For example, Steinmetz (1992) studied the social and economic processes which were seen as bringing about the formation of the English working class. He argued that the working class could only come into being when workers understood the stories of their lives, and of their relation to collective history, in ways that are organized by the category of class (see also Thompson 1972).

Steinmetz also goes some way to distinguishing between different forms of presentational narrative. He separates the 'expert' non-fictional narratives told by official historians, journalists, politicians and so on, from the individual self-narrative, though both are shaped by specific types of ideological structure which he calls the 'collective narrative'. These collective narratives differ from individual accounts of collective groups such as written and oral narratives, 'naturally occurring' stories elicited from other researchers, self-narratives, narratives of external 'others' and anonymous collective narratives (Steinmetz 1992: 490).

Narratologists like Steinmetz have the study of history as the unifying theme in their work, yet come from a number of different theoretical backgrounds. Hence, speaking from a Marxist perspective, Somers (1992) argues that 'social scientists must assume that social reality itself has a narrative structure and... we must attempt to recapture those narratives by narrative means rather than seek universal laws' (cited in Steinmetz 1992: 495). So, though an external social reality is accepted in Somer's historical work, empirical methods are found to be incompatible with the study of social life, whilst the use of the narrative approach can be more fruitful in obtaining an accurate picture of the world and the perceptions of people who inhabit that world.

Taking another view on historical narrative, Hart (1992) has studied nationalist narratives by looking at the role of women in the Greek resistance in the Second World War. The narratives collected showed that the resistance movement for women was communicated not only in nationalistic terms of defending their nation against foreigners but also as political empowerment of certain disempowered groups. Such re-evaluations of history through the use of personal and group narratives lead to the possibility of re-appraising people within different times and cultures. Sewell is aware of the problems of a reliance on narratives to accomplish such tasks and implies that more in-depth work needs to be done to develop the 'historical narrative' perspective. He suggests further probing and analysing of texts, pointing out that writers like Steinmetz and Hart do not actually use narratological techniques 'to take apart a text and show how it works to create specific identities and motivations and to occlude others' (1992: 487). What Sewell implies is that these historians fail to demonstrate specific text-reading strategies which will illuminate the social movements and social processes given in their writings, thus those 'positivistically inclined may feel justified in their scepticism'. The concrete practices of textual analysis need to be outlined and explained clearly to the reader if such narrative work is to be accepted as credible within the social sciences.

Social researchers are increasingly using some sort of 'narrative approach' in the study of social life (for example, Josselson and Lieblich 1993, 1995a), with Josselson (1995) commenting that empathy and narrative should be parts of any research process, though they have been lost by social researchers. These studies are carried out, however, with an unquestioning premise of a structural reality to their enquiries. At no time is there a questioning of the existence of an external social system that we can trace human activity back to. The consequences of this approach are summarized by Chase who notes, 'a major contribution of narrative analysis is *the study of general social phenomena* through a focus on their embodiment in specific life stories' (1995: 2, emphasis added). The limitation of these narrative studies is that they rely on taken-for-granted assumptions about modern society. So whereas Zohar (1995) suggests generalizing from these texts to further our understanding of social life, Denzin (1997) – an 'interpretative ethnographer' – calls for placing of the author's narrative *within the texts,* extracting parts of text that represent cultural and personal interactions, and representing problems of the texts *rather than offering a complete story.* Whilst modernist social science is arguing for the further engagement in qualitative and 'narrative' methods to uncover the social world, interpretative ethnography and social constructionism questions the fundamental possibility of being able to study a 'social world' outside of our own personal conceptions of it. The difference in modernist and post-modernist views of 'narrative study' will now be summarized, illustrating a compromise 'narrative approach' which was utilized by the author with mental health users in Bradford.

2.8 A narrative approach

Denzin (1997) is a chief advocate of the post-structuralist approach to the narrative turn. Following Derrida's (1981) work, he outlines a critique of realist ethnography. A brief summation of his arguments is as follows:

- The research process is not value-free or objective and ethnographers should not make claims as to the nature of the social world without accepting their own interaction with this world. Modernist (structuralist or 'realist') ethnographers have ignored or forgotten how to engage with the subject in the resulting text.
- Realist ethnography is a 'gendered process'; it focuses on and reflects the concerns and attitudes of white, middle-class males and remains emotionally distant from the subject (despite the fact that a certain identity is never possible in the research situation). The ethnographer works with a 'hybrid reality' and needs to be constantly aware of their changing position in research with the subject(s).
- Ethnography is not simply a record of human experience, the ethnographer writes moral tales, tales of agonies, of pain, success and of tragedies of human experience. The stories move people to action; thus the ethnographer has a duty to collect and tell these multiple versions of 'the truth'. Ethnography needs to highlight the emotionality of subjects and anchor text within the world of lived experience.
- 'Realist' ethnographic critiques of other social scientists using different methodologies have served to 'police the boundaries of ethnography, inscribing a proper version of how this form of scientific work should be done' (Denzin 1997: xv). Denzin believes this model to be flawed and inconsequential to representing subjects' narratives. We live in a second-hand world of meanings, there is no way of obtaining direct access to reality; instead 'reality' is mediated by symbolic representations, narrative texts, and by cinematic and televisual structures that stand between the person and the 'real world'.

As a result, Denzin suggests an 'interpretative' (or post-structural) ethnography, where researchers can work in a number of different ways with those researched, including acting as a scribe for the other, writing 'messy' texts (Marcus 1994); co-authoring writing with the other, producing a joint document; producing a purely auto-ethnographic text based on his or her personal experiences; or constructing a 'performance text', with the writer experimenting in new styles of writing.

Denzin clarifies what is meant by writing 'messy' texts. It is a focus 'on those events, narratives, and stories people tell one another as they attempt to make sense of the epiphanies or existential turning point moments in their lives' (1997: xvii). This very much mirrors Gergen's (1994) work on the periods of 'highs' and 'lows' in peoples' narratives. Further, Denzin states that 'messy texts are many cited, open-ended, they refuse theoretical closure, and they do not indulge in abstract analytical theorising. They make the writer a part of the writing project' (1997: xvii). These texts are necessarily multi-voiced and no given interpretation (writer's or subject's) is privileged. It is a rejection of the realist ethnographic narrative that makes claims to textual autonomy and of offering an authentic account of the processes encountered. These messy texts must be well written for both a literary and an academic audience, and should favour emotionality in the stories told to stimulate social critique and social action; it is 'a joining of the personal, the biographical, with the political, the social' (1997: 200).

Some aspects of Denzin's interpretative ethnography is far from new; the Cartesian notion of the objective reality that can be studied to gather social facts about the world was criticized for a large part of the 20th century. As Schutz (1962) has commented, the constructs of the social scientist are second-hand constructs. Smith (1978: 23) explains:

> The phenomena which [the social scientist] studies and seeks to explain are already structured by the interpretations and characterisations of those she studies. That structure is an essential feature of the phenomena, not something added to it which she must strip away to get at 'how things really are'. Moreover the procedures she uses to assemble and interpret her data are not essentially different from those that lay actors use in bringing about the phenomena which becomes her data. What she so uses has already been worked up for purposes which have usually nothing to do with her. In the construction of her data, others have been busy. The process of transforming social action into sociological data must be recognised as a joint, though not ordinarily purposefully concerted, activity.

Many ethnographers have previously recognized the impossibility of divorcing the subject from the researcher and recognized that the research process is, in itself, a form of social interaction. Smith notes that the creation of sociological data is a joint process created from a host of previous and current experiences through dialogue. As Geertz (1983: 6) has remarked, the so-called objective process of sociological 'interpretation' of experiences is a highly relative, contextual concept. He argues that we should reject a cause-and-effect model in favour of orientating ourselves towards 'local knowledge'. The disillusionment with unobtrusive methods and the development of the idea that experience and knowledge lies 'within' people rather than external to them is behind a move towards narrative approaches by many social scientists. For example, Shotter (1989: 133) has remarked that the conduct of research should be 'that of investigating its nature from a position of active involvement in it, rather than contemplative withdrawal from it'. However, most narrative theorists still place an emphasis on the modernist values of analysis and interpretation of people's narratives in their work. As Josselson and Lieblich explain,

> Narrative approaches to understanding bring the researcher more closely into the investigative process than do quantitative and statistical methods. Through narratives we come in contact with our participants as people engaged in the process of interpreting themselves. We work then with what is said and what is not said, within the context in which life is lived and the context of the interview in which words are spoken to represent that life. *We then must decode, recognise, recontextualise, or abstract that life in the interest of reading a new interpretation of the raw data of experience before us.*
>
> (1995b: ix, emphasis added)

This approach to narrative, then, contrasts with a post-structural view which rejects the idea of interpretation and analysis (for example, the 'decoding' of data and so on) as imposing the social scientist's reality on the other and of creating an order on the texts where none exists. The realist approach is one which confuses grammar and experience accounts (Harré 1993: 25): knowledge of personal feelings can only be hinted at through the production of texts, to further 'recontextualize' the narratives is to further lose any semblance of the author's experience and story, and replace it with the researcher's own story instead. For post-structuralists, narratives are part of the process by which an individual constructs a 'reality', and understanding these texts is a way of 'framing' this 'reality'

(Marcus 1994: 567). The texts themselves move back and forth between description, interpretation, and voice; these voices should be highlighted in the analysis, not reduced to generalizations gleaned from small pieces of texts (Denzin 1997: 225). The idea of collecting peoples' narratives to gain a more accurate grasp of experience in a structural context has come from the research of ethnomethodologists, symbolic interactionists and anthropologists, and is informed by social theorists such as Blumer (1969) who has written that 'methods are subservient to [the] world and should be subject to test by it' (cited in Estroff 1981: 37). And further, by writers like Mishler (1986) who has noted that the conventional methods of interviewing have tended to suppress respondents' stories and ignored them in the interpretation of data, which will include stories despite sociologists' attempts to stifle them (cited in Estroff 1981).

Mishler suggests that we impulsively tell stories as an integrated part of human experience; interviewees will tell stories even if they are not encouraged to (see Chase 1995: 1–2). Baumeister and Newman (1994: 676), for example, comment on a prominent researcher who was attempting to do research with successful businessmen to ascertain the key elements of success. The researcher found that his respondents tended to tell stories rather than directly answer the questions asked. At first the researcher thought his respondents were hiding the truth behind these stories, but only later realized that people do not, by and large, express reasons for success in terms of abstract, general principles, 'but instead they tend simply to keep all the relevant information in their memory in narrative terms. The story, rather than the generalisation, was the medium for preserving and communicating information'. This follows the work of earlier qualitative social scientists who found patterns of people's experiences and thoughts would not follow inference, abstraction and the generalization of science but rather narrative forms, hence the recent focus on studying peoples' stories.

Unlike the post-modernist ethnographer, the modernist narrative researcher finds it less problematic to analyse and interpret narrative data and relate the results back to wider social structures and processes. Narrative is first and foremost a *method* which will help social scientists better understand the world through the study of the life experiences of individuals. Josselson (1995) readily sees this as a philosophical idea rooted in hermeneutics; it is a return to the study of experience through empathetic and narrative research. There are recognized problems of 'imagining the real' and the joint process of researcher and subject formulating the narrative together, but not with the ultimate goal of understanding the *wider social context* outside of the individual narrative.

The problems of this approach for structuralist researchers are methodological; for example, how does this 'narrative method' help us find out truths about the world? These writers do not suffer from the ontological insecurities which post-structuralists attempt to tackle. This is illustrated by Josselson's concern to point out the methodological contingencies that are involved in all research: 'we cannot know the real without recognising our own role as knowers', she remarks,

> We take whatever observations we have made of the external world and, making them part of ourselves, interpret them and tell a story about what we believe we know. Empathy and narrative are an inevitable part of all research, whether quantitative or qualitative in design, but these are processes that have been relegated to the shadows in psychology, disowned, disavowed but, like all that is repressed, ever-present.
>
> (1995: 28–9)

In the case of ethnographic narratives, the differences in methodology between the modernist and post-modernist are not insurmountable, the crucial differences are in the analyses of the narratives. A structuralist view of narrative questions the wisdom of neglecting the personal story within social research and academic study as well as the impossibility of framing the research process outside of everyday social interactions of people. The post-structuralist view allows researchers to look at new ways of understanding people and going about the task of collecting social information. As with the structuralist narrative theorists, the link is made between the social scientist and the individual in developing the narrative together. Thus, post-structuralists unashamedly give primacy to the messy text as given and favour emotionality over detachment, asking us to constantly question the research context, how we should go about it and in what form the narrative should appear at the end of the study period.

The author's research with mental health users in Bradford was an attempt to transcend both realist and post-structuralist theoretical approaches to narrative study. That is, a post-structuralist methodology of performing a joint narrative with mental health users, collecting messy texts, was utilized, whilst space was still left for the conceptualization of the resulting texts that temporarily avoided any ideological standpoint. It was possible that the results would show many fractured insights into life perceptions of users or, alternatively, there might be evidence of some unifying themes. The bottom line of the study was to represent and convey user texts accurately, and this called for the suspension of traditional realist assumptions about people and society. In the meantime, it was possible to hold off judgement on whether social processes were constructed or real.

2.9 A definition

Geertz (1983) has commented that though we may start from a particular view of culture, the research work we do with individuals often does not match up to our wider theories. There is often conflict between individual experience of the world and wider theories which are presented to explain the world to us. Thus, Mattingly and Garro see narratives as a vehicle for confronting the contradiction between cultural modes of shared experience and the individual's experience. Giving the example of health care, the malfunctioning body is perceived in Western society as the dichotomy of cause, diagnosis and treatment, but this cultural mode for understanding illness can possibly contradict the individual narrative, leading to a conflict over legitimization of one's suffering if no cause of illness is found. Investigation and legitimization of individual illness narratives will bring about a different viewpoint on the ideas of health care.

Although there may be attempts at modern culture 'speaking to itself', as demonstrated by the use of narrative study within social sciences, there are also some strong boundary divisions which continue to exist. As Geertz (1983: 19–35) has alluded to, different parts of the human sciences have never truly been defined as distinctly different in operation and study, yet there remain some obvious points of departure. This has been witnessed in the different definitions and approaches to narrative study discussed in this chapter, with writers broadly remaining attached to ideological standpoints of their own disciplines. Thus historians and anthropologists explore narratives as a way to further understand particular historical epochs and cultural settings, psychologists and other personality theorists focus on narratives as transmissions of thought processes and cognitions which explain human action and interaction, and sociologists tie narratives to the study of institutions and wider societal processes. The very defining of 'narratives' produces different stories which represent different worldviews within the human sciences. These are, in turn, based on agreed philosophies and acquired rhetoric enshrined within language and professional dialogue.

Through this discussion of different approaches to narrative it is clear that there is no one common definition of narrative and agreed approach to its investigation by social and behavioural scientists. We should not be very surprised at this, as the 'narrative approach' has been a relatively recent addition to the social sciences whereas its use in literature and linguistics has spanned the 20th century (see Plummer 1983). The main theme running through these different approaches is disillusionment with the traditional empirical methods of studying society and individuals, and a philosophical critique of scientific principles. Though debate continues on research methodologies, the protagonists agree on one thing – that 'the myth of detachment' (Rosaldo 1989) from those being studied should be dispensed with. There has been a rejection of the notion that a researcher can remain an objective and neutral collector of information about the social world.

There is a tendency to use the concept of 'narrative' as a broad-based approach to the study of the individual, which can still take a variety of different theoretical directions. The differences that we have seen in the theoretical approaches to the study of narrative by social science theorists is summed up by Harré (1993) with the question, 'are human beings to be taken to be *active agents* using their social knowledge jointly to accomplish certain ends? Or are they *information-processing automata*, the behaviours of which are the effects of casual processes?' (1993: 22, emphases added).

Genette (1988: 13) makes a useful point when he distinguishes between three concepts in narrative discourse: the 'story', which is 'the totality of the narrated events', the 'narrative', which is 'the discourse, oral or written, that narrates [stories]', and the 'narrating', which is 'the real or fictive art that produces discourse', that is the act of recounting the story. And herein lies the problem of untangling the web of narrative, for we may ask where narrative begins and ends. Once a personal 'narrative' is in the public domain is it any longer a 'true' personal narrative or is it an interpretation of personal experience made explicit by social and behavioural scientists? The struggle for definition of 'narrative' reflects this concern. The unifying theme being that narrative is a 'story', the telling of a story, or the investigation of how a story is told. The significance attached to narrative depends on the theoretical standpoint; for example, the narrative may be seen as the uncovering of motivating beliefs of a person (Maynes 1992; Palombo 1992), a creative mode of thought (Baumeister and Newson 1994; Bruner 1986; Heath 1986; Zukier 1986), an explanation for action (Abell 1987; Mattingly and Garro 1994) or forms of public discourse (Gergen 1994).

In reviewing literature on narratives, Sewell (1992) points out that the use of the term 'narrative' signifies a number of different things to different people. It can be 'a universal category of human culture, convention of storytelling, epistemological or ontological assumptions, accounts of life experiences, [or] ideological structures intended to motivate the rank and file of social movements' (1992: 486). Sewell remarks that all these uses may make sense in their own particular context but there may be a dilution of the term 'narrative' taking place. It is argued that there is a need to more formally define the term to give it some 'analytical bite' (1992: 487).

Following Rosenau (1992: xiv), narratives are defined in this book as 'stories' or 'life stories'. This definition is chosen because it offers some clarity on the subject and seeks to demystify a jargon-loaded concept. In essence the definition should be inclusionary rather than exclusionary and, for instance, should allow users to be able to talk freely around life issues, as well as help the researcher to conceptualize the resulting data in a practical manner. For all the theory on narratives, few have outlined a practical methodology and process of analysis (for example, Josselson and Lieblich 1993, 1995a). Thus, a new 'narrative method' was developed by the author, which allowed the users to talk about any issue they wanted to (see Chapter 4). This approach was influenced by Miller (1994) who performed a qualitative study of ten users with 'borderline personality disorders'. Life history narratives were obtained through simply asking the patients to talk about themselves. Miller comments that 'no assumption was made about whether the disorder was central to the patient's experience. What patients chose to tell about themselves and how they chose to do it was left up to them' (1994: 1216). Denzin's 'interpretative ethnography' and other post-structural readings also had an important part in influencing the development of this methodology, especially because Denzin's work places the researcher within the research process rather than outside the collection of the texts. Whilst not offering an exact 'methodology', his writings offer a number of ways in which to conduct text-based research, including writing as a scribe for the 'other' through the collection of 'messy texts' (Marcus 1994: 567).

Despite differences in the use of the 'narratives', there is general agreement amongst those within medical sociology that discovering peoples' narratives offers a more 'humanitarian' way of considering periods of 'illness', rather than following the patterns of disengagement imposed by more 'scientific' views of the body. We have seen this in the work of Baumeister and Newman (1994: 676) who claim that it is the story rather than the *generalization* which is the medium through which people present and communicate information. With mental health users this means that the re-establishment of 'personhood' and 'citizenship' within society may be seen as more significant to recovery than the understanding of their particular 'disorder'. Narrative study can allow for the unravelling of these complex issues (Barham and Hayward 1991: 3).

2.10 Conclusion

The narrative approach used in this book derives from the questioning of the primacy of certain narratives (such as those of professional groups) over other narratives. Building on social constructionist concepts of peoples' identities being reproduced over time through collected life stories together with Denzin's 'interpretative ethnographic' approach, a central aim of this book is to conceptualize psychiatric user life stories with the minimum of interpretation by the author. That is, the author will 'act as a scribe for the other' (see Denzin 1997: 231–49) to build an understanding of peoples' constructions of reality rather than producing 'the truth' of psychiatric user experiences. The purpose of taking a narrative approach allows for user stories to be recorded with the minimum of intervention and interpretation from outside forces. Given the limited number of studies that have given primacy to user voices within the mental health system, this alternative approach can emancipate both the researcher and the user. Even if the power relationship in an interview situation remains unbalanced, social scientists must still recognize and attempt to deal with this situation to increase user/interviewee input and thus peoples' ability to communicate their views.

This chapter has illustrated the rise of the 'narrative' concept within the behavioural sciences and the humanities. Interest in personal narratives has been heightened by the influences of post-modern writings as well as disillusionment with the currently available research methodologies. It has also been shown, however, that the term 'narrative' can mean different things to different writers, and subsequent definitions reflect this. It is further confused through some writers introducing new theoretical propositions which see narrative study as integral to new forms of knowledge (such as social constructionism), whilst other social scientists use narratives as a new form of methodology which can be integrated into their current ideological positions. Particularly post-modernist thinking has criticized the use of Western science as a form of knowledge production, constructed by and increasingly reliant on language and narrative forms to legitimate its activities. In the social sciences, interpretative ethnography has called on researchers to look at alternative ways of exploring the narratives of those researched and presenting them to the reader.

The issues of re-constructing a 'social reality' through our experience has been commented on by Elias (1991: 6) who notes,

> We try to reconstruct in thought what we experience each day in reality [and] we find, as with a jigsaw puzzle the pieces of which will not form a whole picture, that gaps and fissures are constantly forming in our train of thought.

Narrative study allows exploration of this 'jigsaw puzzle' and further reflection on the individual. Chapter 3 describes the development of crisis intervention programmes within psychiatry. It focuses particularly on the Bradford Home Treatment Service and their workings with mental health users, which utilized alternative models of care including a narrative approach. The mental health users from this home treatment project forms half the sample for the narrative research described later in this book.

3
Crisis Intervention and Home Treatment

> I just assumed once you got in that state you were whipped off to hospital.
>
> (Helen)

3.1 Summary

As part of the transfer of resources from inpatient to community-based care, there has been a marked increase in varieties of 'crisis intervention' service in the past few years. Brimblecombe (2001: 5) remarks that some of these services provide extended hours and have 'an explicit or implicit aim of reducing acute admissions to psychiatric wards'. A popular form of service that has been piloted in many countries has been the 'home treatment' or 'home care' programmes. There have been a plethora of studies comparing hospital treatment with home treatment programmes over the past 40 years which have repeatedly demonstrated that home-based care offers a better of quality of service to users and is cost-effective (for an overview of the research see, for example, Orme and Cohen 2001; Smyth and Hoult 2000). Recent government reviews in the United States and the United Kingdom have recognized the importance of offering crisis intervention services to avoid hospital admission (Department of Health 1999, 2007; President's New Freedom Commission on Mental Health 2003). At the time of writing, however, there is still a marked variation in the both the breadth and depth of crisis provision offered from area to area (Brimblecombe 2001; Hogan *et al.* 1997).

This Chapter investigates the background and development of crisis intervention services, before exploring the foundation, development and progress of the Bradford Home Treatment Service in the United Kingdom. This alternative to hospitalization operated successfully in

Bradford for 7 years and was given 'Mental Health Beacon' status for 3 years by the NHS (see National Health Service 2002). There was national media coverage on the workings and philosophy of this home treatment team, particularly focusing on their 'radical' user-centred approach to care (for example, see BBC 2002; James 2000). Falling into line with current mental health policy, the Bradford Home Treatment Service is now the 'Bradford Crisis Resolution Home Treatment Service'. The significance of this change will also be addressed. The author worked closely with the Bradford Home Treatment Service in the early years of its operation (1996–1999). The narratives from a number of users from this service will be reproduced later in this book and compared with those users who received hospital treatment.

3.2 Crisis intervention

Since the 1950s and 1960s the idea of 'preventative psychiatry' has gathered pace within the field of mental health, expanding public consciousness of the everyday afflictions of stress, worry, disturbance, depression, neuroses, and so on. If not understood and 'treated', these disturbances could possibly lead to more serious mental illnesses. Caplan (1964) was a key writer on the subject and influenced the development of 'crisis intervention' services. He identified three phases of the 'crisis': the first phase is the rise in tension where a person realizes something is wrong; the second is the point of crisis, where a person's internal resources are exhausted and overcome; and the third represents the resolution of crisis through either growth or stagnation. According to Caplan, the second phase – when people are most open to suggestion – is the appropriate time to intervene with therapy. From this initial concept of intervening in a person's crisis other writers developed the definition further. Renshaw (1989) described the concept as providing appropriate help quickly to clients with identifiable psychological crises, with the aim of returning clients to their pre-crisis level of functioning. Appropriate intervention depends on mental health personnel identifying who is in crisis, what stage the crisis has reached and what kind of help is needed.

With the help of such writers in the 1960s, crisis intervention extended further the services available in the community for people with mental health problems, usually taking a more focused approach to those in need and, in this way, separating themselves from aftercare and outpatient services. Newton (1989) described three basic ways in which crisis intervention services could operate: they could run parallel to current services with referrals coming from the same sources, they might be integrated into local mental health provision with one point of entry for clients, or a crisis service might target one particular population and select its referrals in terms of their suitability to the treatment offered. Most importantly, Newton added that there was no blueprint for a crisis intervention service and that local resources, demands and needs would influence the development of a service and how it works. Thus, in a survey by Hogan *et al.* (1997) of English Health Authorities in the 1990s, it was found that 16 per cent of health authorities purchase no crisis services at all, 31 per cent purchase crisis response, intervention, early or rapid-response services, 15 per cent purchase home support, home treatment, community support or community respite, 15 per cent purchase a combination of the two, and the rest purchase other types of ad hoc services. Of most concern was Hogan's comment that 'a fair proportion of all [crisis] services are "pilot" schemes or are temporary for one reason or another and do not endure as an integrated part of mental health provision' (1997: 3). It can therefore be seen that, in the 1990s, many parts of the United Kingdom were attempting to develop some sort of crisis response service, yet it was also debatable as to how sustainable such projects were going to be. This uncertainty was to affect the fate of the Bradford Home Treatment Service.

Part of the problem of the development of crisis services during this period may have been to do with the definition of 'crisis intervention' itself. Renshaw (1989) stated that the term meant different things to different people, for example, some advocates of crisis intervention believed its role was to avoid hospital admission, whilst others (such as Bengelsdorf *et al.* 1993) were of the opinion that, as well as supporting clients in their own homes, crisis intervention should regard hospitalization as a necessary and acceptable part of therapy in some cases. Both views can be considered part of crisis intervention. As Hobbs (1984: 32) remarked,

> There is very little consensus, even among practitioners, as to what constitutes crisis intervention. A variety of techniques are applied in a variety of settings to a whole variety of problems, by practitioners with a variety of skills and qualifications, and with a variety of aims.

Renshaw noted further that just because a service called itself a 'crisis intervention service' did not mean it was practising 'crisis intervention'; a rapid response did not mean that it was applying crisis theory.

Despite these concerns, the logic of community care demands 'rapid response' to requests for help, with care to be given as close to home as possible and with the minimum of hospitalization. It has been argued by Burti and Tansella (1995) that acute home-based care typically meets these requirements. In acute situations, hospital provides treatment and refuge for patients, and respite for families, but will usually be of short duration. 'In contrast, a community treatment team provides ongoing care, and is available at all times for emergencies. The team's readiness to respond to early worries of the patient and/or family may even *prevent* emergencies' (1995: 277, emphasis original).

Developed out of community care legislation, Bean and Mounser (1993) describe the emergence of the modern multi-disciplinary team which has taken the dominant form of 'sectorization' of mental health care. This 'sectorization' espouses the treatment of the patient by community psychiatric teams, the principle being that – whether the person is in the community or in hospital – they are dealt with by the same people and 'continuity of care' is ensured. The multi-disciplinary teams are organized in sectors of around 100,000 people with the same consultant being responsible for the patient over the length of their treatment. As Bean and Mounser point out, 'sectorisation by itself is not a system of "community care", but the administrative means by which it can be achieved' (1993: 64). As a general rule, each sector has two consultant psychiatrists allocated to it, each with a multi-disciplinary team of workers (usually including social workers, community psychiatric nurses, a general practitioner, senior nursing staff and occupational therapists), who will deal with users both as inpatients and as outpatients. Some consultants have specializms in certain areas (such as alcohol and drugs, or psychotherapy) and will still cover the whole district. These consultants are usually hospital-based, though some have moved into the community. This system of sectorization was reflected in the Bradford district in the mid-1990s, which had five sectors, each with its own team and local population to serve.

3.3 Home treatment

For the purpose of profiling forms of home-based service, 'home treatment' is defined as any formal psychiatric service where mental health workers attend the home as part of an intensive therapeutic intervention. The service does not necessarily have to be a stated 'alternative' to hospitalization or 'crisis intervention service', although these are the preferred options in many cases. While there are many different forms of 'home treatment' in existence the term is mostly taken to refer to services which provide (a) 24-hour availability and (b) intensive home visiting by mental health workers. These services are sometimes called 'home-based care services' and both terms are used interchangeably here.

The first reported service of this kind was established in Amsterdam, Holland, in the early 1930s (Querido 1968). The premise was that rehabilitation should be a social process which is accomplished in the community itself. Establishing the ideal of home treatment as an 'alternative' to hospitalization, Querido found that 70 per cent of referrals for hospitalization could be handled in this way. Besides being a form of management, the home visit was important in being able to study the dynamics of the mental illness crisis in situ. Mickle has stated that this programme became the prototype for community home visiting services (1963: 379). As early as 1949, home visiting programmes were established in Nottingham (MacMillan 1958) and, later, in Worthing (Carse *et al.* 1958), both in the United Kingdom. The advantages cited in these schemes were a more accurate evaluation, establishment of a better relationship with the patient and family, and the discussion of alternative treatment where possible (Mickle 1963).

With the number of hospitalized patients reaching record highs in many Western countries by the 1950s, Burti and Tansella (1995) note the need arising for comprehensive care of discharged patients and expanding the practice of home visiting, for both crisis intervention and follow-up. 'Home visiting', comment the authors, 'became an everyday routine for community psychiatric nurses (CPNs), since the 1950s in England (Woof *et al.* 1988), and from the 1960s in France (Fournaise 1988; Maurin 1990), Russia (Singer *et al.* 1969) and in Italy (Jervis 1975)' (1995: 276–7). Yet it is also noted that 'house calls' by psychiatrists remained rare during this period (Burti and Tansella 1995: 277). This situation had changed by the 1980s, where Chiu and Primeau (1991) note a more positive attitude of psychiatrists in the United Kingdom towards making home visits than their colleagues in the United States.

Some early cases of home-based treatment projects were reported in North America in the 1950s and 1960s. Meyer *et al.* (1967) reported on a home treatment service operating as an alternative to hospitalization in Boston, which had been established in 1957. Consisting of a psychiatrist, a registered nurse, a social worker and an occupational therapist (an early version of the multi-disciplinary team), the service was able to divert more than half the cases referred to hospital. The authors found that the home treatment service was more effective in maintaining patients in the community through the use of pharmacological therapy and interventions in the social and familial structures around the patient. Early attempts were also made to involve non-medical professionals (for example, clergy and welfare workers) in the treatment.

Projects such as Meyer *et al.*'s (1967) and Chiu and Primeau's (1991) Mobile Crisis Unit in New York City were influenced by the European alternatives to hospital treatment as well as the flow of interpretative psychiatric theory, crisis intervention and the developments in community psychiatry. Given America's burgeoning fiscal crisis with respect to mental health care, the reports of alternatives to hospitalization appeared very attractive. Singer *et al.*'s (1969) first-hand experiences of the home visiting models in the Soviet Union and Holland – reported in the *American Journal of Psychiatry* – showed how home visits avoided the need for hospitalization in all but a handful of cases and allowed more flexibility in local mental health teams' ability to deal with individual periods of mental distress.

A number of home-based projects were developed in the 1970s, which refined further the goals of home treatment and the advantages of this approach. At the time, Chapell and Daniels (1970, 1972) noted the objections raised to this approach: the projects were expensive in terms of time and money; they could be difficult and dangerous; they possibly interfered with treatment by breeding dependency or 'acting out'; and they increased the burden on the family and community. The authors found from their own home visiting project in Chicago, however, that these objections were more internal resistance than external reality. The psychiatrists concluded that home visiting was possible and safe; that it may bridge isolation, alienation and hopelessness found in deprived areas; that it may enlist the support of family and friends, which could not be encountered in the office setting; that it may be helpful in treating violent or paranoid patients and in avoiding the disruption of hospital treatment; and that it may be a way of bridging cultural gaps and building a basis for trust between doctor and patient in which the patient can play an active part.

Mosher *et al.* (1975) took the possibility of patient participation a step further in California, with a 'home-like facility' for schizophrenics – called 'Soteria' – being attended by non-professionals. The study was one of the first to compare home-based treatment with an institutionalized form of mental health care. Similarly, Coates *et al.* (1976) compared home treatment in Vancouver with hospital treatment and found home treatment cheaper, more efficient and a preferred option for users and relatives. Polak and Kirby (1976) found that their 'total community care system' in Denver (which included a home treatment service) reduced the need for inpatient beds to less than one in 100,000. Bringing together earlier ideas from home treatment projects of involving the patient, family and community in the provision of care, Polak and Kirby encouraged citizen participation and community control through eliminating staff offices and focusing on the 'real life settings' of the client and family.

Given the cynicism with which psychiatry had greeted community policies in general, it is unsurprising that such projects were – and to some degree, still are – regarded with scepticism. A critique at the time was that no standardized research had been carried out to measure home treatment as an effective and efficient alternative to hospitalization. The first such study was completed by Test and Stein (1980) in Wisconsin, Madison. Their 'Training in Community Living' programme (a total in-community programme) was compared with standard hospital and aftercare, using a randomized procedure to divide patients in crisis into two groups. The staff were specifically trained to promote daily activities in the community for the experimental (that is, home treatment) group. The results showed no more burden on the family or the community than did the traditional approach, and a greater level of satisfaction. Test and Stein's approach has been replicated in Australia (see Hoult *et al.* 1983) and England (see Muijen *et al.* 1992). Other studies on home treatment have been carried out in North America, Europe, India, Brazil and Australia since the 1980s. These research projects have, likewise, shown that home treatment compares well to hospitalization (see Orme and Cohen 2001) and can be equally effective with adolescents (for example, Seelig *et al.* 1992) and older users (for example, Rosenzweig *et al.* 1996).

Various ad hoc home treatment projects have developed in the United Kingdom over the past 30 years. For example, a crisis intervention team was set up in 1979 in Lewisham, south London, which offered psychiatric intervention in the community for people who would otherwise have needed hospital admission (see Tufnell *et al.* 1985). In 1981, Tyrer *et al.* (1989) set up a diversionary psychiatric scheme in Nottingham with the idea of offering treatment as close to people's homes as possible. Both projects found that treatment had to alter in the home setting and that 'psychosocial' interventions (i.e. a mixture of social and psychological interventions) were preferred to strictly medical ones. Admissions to hospital fell in both cases. However, it was not until the establishment of the Maudsley Daily Living Programme (DLP) in Southwark, London, that home treatment came to be seen as a serious option by health authorities and professionals. This project replicated Test and Stein's programme to assess its applicability to the British mental health care system. The programme provided 24-hour care, case management at the site of breakdown, brief in-patient admission if necessary, assertive follow-up, encouragement and maintenance of daily living skills, support and education of the people seen as important to the patient's well-being and advocacy if necessary. Though the DLP had its problems, the results showed again a fall in hospital admissions, a cheaper service and more satisfaction from carers and clients (see Audini *et al.* 1994; Marks *et al.* 1988, 1994; Muijen *et al.* 1992). As Hogan *et al.* (1997) noted above, many crisis intervention services have been set up for limited periods and/or as 'pilot projects', and home treatment services are no exception. It is therefore of little surprise that the longest running home treatment service in the United Kingdom is said to be North Birmingham's home treatment service (see Sashidharan and Smyth 1992) – a programme that is less than 20 years old.

Though the programmes had been in existence for longer, home treatment projects were given professional credibility through crisis intervention theory in the 1960s and successful controlled studies in the 1980s. As an alternative to hospitalization for mental heath users in acute crisis, home treatment has been repeatedly demonstrated as cost-effective and a better quality of service for both users and carers. 'Home treatment' or 'home-based care' has also allowed psychiatry to innovate with new technologies, experiment with the community and extend its working practices. At the same time, there is also the possibility of challenging traditional psychiatric philosophies and modes of treatment. Treating the patient outside the institution can lead to new insights for the care worker, and resistance to biomedical solutions can evolve. This will be illustrated with reference to the formation, philosophy and early workings of the Bradford Home Treatment Service in the following section.

3.4 Background

In 1990s Britain, very high acute psychiatric bed occupancy rates were being reported in many parts of the country. This was particularly the case in London and other inner city areas. Health Trusts were being faced with a demand for more acute psychiatric places. However, in its report 'Finding a Place', the Audit Commission identified the vicious circle in which it was difficult to develop community services because of the pressure on hospital beds where most health service resources were tied up (Audit Commission 1994). The commission commented that 'all authorities should be planning how they are to break this vicious circle'.

Bradford, a northern city with a large immigrant population and high levels of social deprivation, was experiencing similar problems: a low number of beds (84) available at the local psychiatric hospital for a population of approximately 457,500. By the mid-1990s, bed utilization rates in Bradford had become extremely high and there was a felt need to develop more acute services outside of the psychiatric hospital. Additionally, a very active user movement had developed in Bradford and the surrounding area which was calling for alternative forms of acute provision to hospital and the development of crisis services (Bailey 1994). A person of significance here was the Chief Executive of the local Health Trust, who came from a mental health background himself and was an enthusiastic supporter of home treatment services. Inspired by the success of other British home treatment projects such as the North Birmingham Home Treatment Service (see Sashidharan and Smyth 1992), he introduced cost savings across the local health services which allowed for the development of a new community service. Thus, in 1995 a decision was reached by the provider trust and the health authority to expand acute provision by developing a home treatment service.

A period of preparation followed, bringing together all interested parties from the local health and social services to assess the feasibility of putting such an operation into practice. This in turn led to the formation of an Advisory Group representing all the affected parties and to the initial recruitment of an Administrator, a Nursing Manager and a Consultant. Soon afterwards an Operational Policy was agreed by the Advisory Group in January 1996. A full home treatment team was added to the three initial recruits. These consisted of one Clinical Medical Officer (CMO), 11 Community Health Nurses (reflecting all major nursing grades from Assistant Community Psychiatric Nurse to Team Leader), two Social Work Assistants and one Approved Social Worker (funded by the local Social Services department), one Community Psychiatric Nurse (CPN) responsible for liaison with the Local Mental Health Resource Centre (a quarter-time post which was later discontinued) and one Service User Development Worker (working four days a week). The multi-disciplinary home treatment team, therefore, started with 20 members of staff. The Bradford Home Treatment Service began formal operations in February 1996. Initially the service was targeted at the Ashgrove sector – the largest of five catchments areas in Bradford – which covered the southwest of the city as well as parts of the city centre.

3.5 Philosophy

Bradford Home Treatment Service's Operational Policy stated that the project was created 'to provide a high quality community based service which provides an alternative to hospital for individuals with acute and severe mental health problems' (1996: 2). Though a definition of 'acute and severe mental health problems' was not suggested in this document, reference was made in the 'acceptance' criteria for patients, that people must need 'intensive input' which would otherwise require 'admission to hospital'. As to what 'a high quality community based service' might look like, reference was made under a section entitled 'values'. These values of the service were said to consist of a partnership with service users and carers, non-coercive interventions, a negotiation with clients regarding assessment and treatment issues, non-discriminatory practice, a commitment to the continual development of home treatment, and a commitment to promoting good practice and high professional standards. Though some of these values might have sounded like the usual rhetoric of mental health-speak, there were some interesting interpretative/critical psychiatric strains observed. For instance, under 'non-coercive interventions' it was stated that 'the service will avoid the use of stigmatising labels', as well as offer care, support and assistance which might be challenging to the user but should not silence the users' ideas or undermine their confidence (1996: 24). Further, it was written that the 'clients are to be involved in "making sense" of their own experience' (a distinctive nod in the direction of narrative psychiatry). In this way, the service was making some quite radical proposals for the way it wanted to work with users and carers. Like a number of the home treatment staff, the Nursing Manager had become quite disillusioned with health practices and saw the service as a way she could stay within nursing and challenge traditional practices. She commented on how she saw the new service developing:

> I think we should be working quite differently. So I think one of our objectives should be that we try and challenge what's been done and try and work differently. I think that's the thing that's most difficult... to do: to not just reproduce what's at [the psychiatric hospital] in the community. So I think we should be providing a high quality but quite innovative service, so we are doing different things, not just churning out what people could have received in hospital.

A three-week training period was carried out with all the team members, including lengthy discussions of how the service would work in practice. As the Operational Policy was quite broad, this allowed the team to develop the service together rather than having the service directly imposed on them. Consequently, the Operational Policy document was revised several times by the team, though the main themes were not radically altered. The Operational Policy (1996) stated that the team would work together in an egalitarian way, all members of the team should be encouraged to share their viewpoint with others, members should be respected for their skills, experiences and opinions, and there should be a move away from the hierarchical grading system used in nursing towards the group as the decision-making body. Similarly, the philosophy for working with users respected their point of view and encouraged staff to understand and work with users in distress. Alternatives to medication were to be facilitated and hospitalization would be discouraged. The home treatment staff translated this broadly as a move away from the 'medical model' towards a 'social model' of care.

A key element of the Bradford Home Treatment Service was the orientation towards a 'user perspective'. The recruited Service User Development Worker was an ex-user of psychiatric services and had been active in local user groups. This person was considered a full member of the team and his work included encouraging user involvement with the team as well as ensuring that the practices of the team were genuinely 'user-sensitive'. This role developed in significance over time, with Relton and Thomas (2002: 347) later commenting that the Service User Development Worker was responsible for addressing issues of power between professional and client:

> [The Service User Development Worker] ... participates in review meetings at which clients' care is discussed, provides training and information to the team grounded in the growing body of research and other writings by mental health service users/survivors, and plays an active part in the local (and national) user/survivor movement. He visits home treatment clients from time to time, for example if someone wants to talk about the politics of mental health or opportunities for volunteering in Bradford, or if they simply want to talk to another user. However, his role is primarily about supporting the team to develop and maintain a non-medical philosophy. The success of the service is fundamentally related to this philosophy of care.

Pat Bracken (2002), the original consultant with the Bradford Home Treatment Service, strongly supported this philosophy and further clarified the team's approach:

> The home treatment service attempts to work with a 'needs led' approach and does not, for the most part, seek to diagnose the service user's problems in a medical way. At times, a medical diagnosis is necessary and important, as when there is a suspicion that organic factors might be affecting the person's condition... The point is that the team's interventions are not guided by psychiatric diagnoses and theories. Psychotropic drugs are used and occasionally the administration of medication becomes a priority. However, these drugs are generally used on a symptomatic basis and not with the belief that they are curing a psychiatric 'disease' of some sort... [We] believe that the benefits of these drugs have been exaggerated in the psychiatric literature and in the claims made by the pharmaceutical industry... The home treatment team is also concerned with the down-side of psychiatric interventions and treatments and is particularly wary of the longer term effects of these drugs... Admissions are more often driven by social problems and poor housing than by the nature of the psychiatric disturbance as such. Working outside the hospital and with an alternative perspective on the nature of depression and despair means that different ways of engaging with individuals in distress become available. We attempt to encounter depression as a 'site of struggle' rather than as an illness, and offer to struggle for a solution alongside the individual in question. It is my belief that this opens up different ways of understanding the reasons behind depression and different ways of going forward.

From my own observations of the Bradford Home Treatment Service during this period it is fair to say that Pat Bracken attempted to challenge the prior beliefs of (primarily) the psychiatric staff on the team, whilst not asserting specific ways in which work with users *must* be carried out. Consequently, Bracken notes that whilst the Bradford Home Treatment Service did not start out to be 'post-psychiatry' (see Section 1.4), in practice it followed many elements of that philosophy in working with users. At the very least, the philosophy of the Bradford Home Treatment Service was cited as 'non-psychiatric' (Bracken 2001).

3.6 Practice

From the beginning, the Bradford Home Treatment Service provided input on a 24-hour, seven days a week basis. Medical input was provided by the team's full-time CMO. The decision to admit patients or to refer to home treatment was made by the sector consultant (based at the local psychiatric hospital) during normal working hours and by the duty consultant out of hours. Patients were visited as often as necessary, sometimes two to three times per day. Regular contact by telephone was established and, if needed, patients were given the use of a mobile phone for the length of their stay on the home treatment service.

The first year is always going to be the hardest for a new team and it is to the credit of both team members and other professionals involved that most realized this; the notes and interviews carried out by the author during this period are full of references to 'teething difficulties', 'finding their feet' and 'development issues'. Nevertheless, it was evident that the cohesion and morale of the team could easily be affected by changes in the wider infrastructure as well as internal perceptions of the team's performance.

For the first few months of operation there were few referrals to the Bradford Home Treatment Service, the work was slow. By the summer, however, home treatment were near to filling their maximum number of 12 client places and the hospital recorded just two admissions from home treatment's sector (Ashgrove) in July 1996, the lowest on record. Unfortunately, it was at this time that the sympathetic consultant for the Ashgrove sector left the hospital. In her place came a succession of locum consultants who were unfamiliar with home treatment and felt it unsuitable in many cases. The reasons for this attitude can be summarized as a lack of knowledge of what the purpose of home treatment was (many locums saw it as an avenue for early discharge rather than as an alternative to hospital) and a highly medicalized idea of what appropriate treatment for mental health users should consist of. Consequently, home treatment referrals declined whilst hospital admissions increased towards the end of 1996. An evaluation report of the first year of operations (see Cohen 1997a) showed that home treatment had reduced hospital admissions from the Ashgrove sector by 25 per cent of the previous year and that the quality of service to users was felt to be much better than hospital care. The cost of service (per 'bed day'), however, was higher compared to the hospital. This was due to the low turnover of users and the low number of client spaces available on home treatment. Inappropriate referrals (that is, not 'acute' or 'severe' cases) were also highlighted as a problem for the Bradford Home Treatment Service (Cohen 1997a).

Mindful of the Bradford Home Treatment Service's need to be seen as a serious alternative to hospital and the damage the current situation was doing to local credibility, the service's consultant negotiated the expansion of the service from the Ashgrove sector to all five Bradford sectors in January 1997, meaning that the service could take referrals from across the city. The maximum number of users the service would accept at one time was provisionally 15 but the total sometimes got closer to 20. The expansion of the catchment area had the positive effect of seeing the number of users rapidly increase and demonstrated to other consultants the effectiveness of the service in redirecting users away from hospital treatment. Working at an optimal level allowed the team to further assess the nature of the service and how to maximize efficiency within team and inter-agency interactions.

By the summer of 1997 a new sympathetic consultant (Phil Thomas) had been employed by the Health Trust to cover home treatment's original Ashgrove sector. At this point the service ceased its city-wide operations and went back to working mainly in this sector, additionally taking a limited number of referrals from a neighbouring sector where the hospital consultant was positive towards the service's input. Due to the closeness of the home treatment and sector consultants' working relationships, when users entered the psychiatric system at these referral points preference was given to the Bradford Home Treatment Service. An evaluation report produced after a further 12 months showed home treatment provided a better quality of service, with 81 per cent of users surveyed finding home treatment 'better' or 'much better' than hospital overall, compared to only 12 per cent finding hospital 'better' or 'much better' than home treatment (Cohen 1999a). Performing further interviews with users who had received hospital treatment only, less than half found hospital to be a positive experience (see Cohen 1999a, 1999b). The Bradford Home Treatment Service also maintained a reduced number of users in hospitals and was found to be cost-effective (Cohen 1999a).

3.7 The end of the Bradford Home Treatment Service

Following the end of the evaluation period of the Bradford Home Treatment Service, in 2000 I wrote the following summary of the service:

> Despite political maneuverings, a current re-sectorisation of the city, and a degree of staff turnover, the production of the final evaluation report [Cohen 1999a] together with the influence of key players and current government policy initiatives have helped to further secure the Bradford Home Treatment Service's place within the local community mental health care system. The service has been nominated for a number of national awards for good practice, and received a number of grants to further programme initiatives. With local re-sectorisation currently taking place, it looks likely that two further home treatment teams will be created within the Bradford area as a direct result of the success of the first project.
>
> (Cohen 2001)

With hindsight, this was an over-optimistic assessment. Following the historical pattern of most home treatment projects, the Bradford Home Treatment Service did not last 10 years in its original form. The service was subsequently merged into a new Crisis Resolution Team (CRT) – the Bradford Crisis Resolution Home Treatment Service – becoming a different form of crisis intervention in the process. The reasons for this change can be briefly summarized as a change in personnel, problems with the original philosophy of the Bradford Home Treatment Service and, above all, a change in governmental directives for mental health care in the United Kingdom.

Through personal correspondence (2007) with the former Nursing Manager of the Bradford Home Treatment Service it is clear that the sustainability of the service was, in part, reliant on the retention of key dynamic personnel. When, for example, the sympathetic Chief Executive of the Bradford Health Trust stepped down, the Bradford Home Treatment Service lost a powerful ally. Despite my positive evaluation of the service (see Cohen 1999a), the Bradford Home Treatment Service was now open to new threats and had to work harder to justify their position in the local mental health care system. Antagonism from other parts of the health care system at the money spent on the new service had been aggravated by the perceived 'anti-psychiatry' philosophy of the team (see Cohen 2001). Without support from senior management, the Bradford Home Treatment Service was exposed to further criticism. All the talk of 'post-psychiatry' and a 'needs-led approach' backfired on the service. The former Nursing Manager explained to me recently (personal correspondence 2007) that 'things got so bad we stopped talking about a "philosophy" altogether'. By 2003, the original Bradford Home Treatment Service team was also breaking up. As new staff members joined, the day-to-day workings of the team began to change: there was less discussion around alternative approaches to treatment, less training days. The consultants Bracken and Thomas eventually left the Bradford Home Treatment Service for positions elsewhere, as did the Nursing Manager. In 2001, the UK government unveiled plans for the creation of 'Crisis Resolution Teams' (CRTs) around the country, with the corresponding press release noting that, 'pilot schemes in areas including Newcastle, Bradford and Camden, have already found that early intervention can prevent 85 per cent of patients from having to receive hospital treatment' (cited in Surgerydoor 2002). It was both a positive recognition of the value of home treatment and other forms of crisis intervention and the beginning of the end for the Bradford Home Treatment Service. Like all public sector operations in the United Kingdom, the health service has a responsibility to meet specific governmental targets on indicators of cost, quality of service, staffing levels, turnover of customers, customer satisfaction, amount of provision, and so on. The fulfilment of these targets is assessed on behalf of the government by the Healthcare Commission. The Healthcare Commission (2005) stated that the characteristics of the CRTs will be:

- a multi-disciplinary team;
- capacity to offer intensive support at service users' homes;
- staff in frequent contact with service users, often seeing them at least once on each shift;
- provision of intensive contact over a short period of time; and
- staff stay involved until the problem is resolved.

Though these characteristics are similar to those of home treatment, the reality of the services can be quite different. The Nursing Manager of the new Bradford Crisis Resolution Home Treatment Service (personal correspondence 2007) – who was also a member of staff with the Bradford Home Treatment Service – conferred that certain aspects of the service had changed. Firstly, the number of clients on the service is, 'about ten times more than the Bradford Home Treatment Service dealt with' and client turnover is much quicker. Users are with the service for 'usually three to four weeks'. The CRT employs around 30 staff to manage a local sector population of around 300,000 (a similar ratio to that of the Bradford Home Treatment Service). The positive effects of the CRT are that they reach many more clients than the Bradford Home Treatment Service did. Consequently, they are also reaching government targets for the number of clients that access the service. Obviously, the negative side of this new CRT is that the team has limited time with each service user. The Nursing Manager openly stated that the philosophy of the CRT was quite different to that of the Bradford Home Treatment Service: there is less time spent with individual users and this can mean that treatment is sometimes reduced to simply dealing with the user's medications. There are now over 335 CRTs across the United Kingdom. This is now the standard response to crisis intervention in the country, yet the significance of the loss of Bradford Home Treatment Service will be illustrated in the analysis chapters that follow. Fundamentally, the Bradford Home Treatment Service offered users a different way of understanding their distress and this has partly been lost under the logic of governmental policy.

3.8 Conclusion

Home treatment services are a part of an ill-defined community mental health care package formed out of social, political and professional shifts in concepts of society, the individual and mental health. In this context it is a testament to the strength of the psychiatric discipline – as a professional and political body – that it has not only weathered these changes but expanded its apparatus into the community (see Rose 1989, 1999). Though the psychiatric profession has had its discontents from both inside and outside the discipline, it remains unified on the crucial issues of the retention of biomedical practices and the need for institutional care. This model may be reinforced through the development of CRTs in the United Kingdom, or the CRTs may be able to develop more socially orientated models of treatment in the long term. Chapter 4 explores the practical processes involved in collecting and analysing hospital and home treatment user narratives.

4
Methods

> Do you not have a set agenda of questions that you follow as such, then?
>
> (Michael)

4.1 Summary

Previous chapters have investigated theories of mental illness, the development of psychiatry, the rise of narrative approaches in psychiatry and the humanities and the development of crisis intervention programmes as rapid-response alternatives to institutional care. It has been shown that theories, treatment and care for the mentally ill continue to be debated. This is why I utilize a narrative approach in researching users of mental health services – we cannot be sure what exactly mental illness is, therefore the research searches for answers within user stories and experiences. The problems and the issues encountered in carrying this narrative method through from theory to practice will be described and explored in this chapter. How the study was conducted in practice as well as the difficulties in achieving the original goals of presenting and understanding user narratives will be described. The research compares the user narratives of people who experienced hospitalization with those who were cared for by the Bradford Home Treatment Service (BHTS), which acted as a new alternative to hospitalization. As the author was already employed to evaluate the BHTS and was in contact with psychiatrists and other health professionals on a regular basis, access to the mental health users for such narrative interviews was easier than it would otherwise have been, though gaining access to the names of people who had been in hospital became more difficult.

4.2 The home treatment sample

Between August 1997 and July 1998, two users who had been discharged from the BHTS every month were chosen randomly for interview. On discharge from home treatment every user received a letter from the home treatment psychiatrists mentioning the possibility of being selected for interview and encouraging them to take part in the research if this was the case (see Appendix A.1). When a user was randomly chosen for interview, a letter was sent by the author explaining the research process and asking for the possibility of an interview (see Appendix A.2). The letters were also translated into Punjabi and people were given the option of a bilingual researcher to try to maximize the number of positive responses from ethnic minority users (the largest second language for inner-city Bradford residents is Punjabi, often preferred by first-generation immigrants from Pakistan). Users were given the option of telephoning or returning a response to the author via a reply-paid envelope. The letter stated that if the author had not heard from the user in a week's time he would try contacting them by telephone. Given it was a random sample, we had to try to maximize positive responses to this request as we could not re-sample unless we had received *no response* after trying every avenue to contact the user.

Most home treatment users did not respond by returning the reply slip, so they were telephoned by the author. If no response was obtained by telephoning, the user was usually visited in person at their house for a possible response, and if no response was attained from calling in person, another letter would be sent as a reminder and further telephoning was carried out. This process was made harder if the user was not on the telephone (as was true in a number of cases). A schedule was formed on a separate database to keep track of who was outstanding for a response, how many letters, telephone calls and so on there had been and over what period of time. The usual cut-off point was after three months when users had been telephoned, visited and reminded of the study. Only then would a re-sample take place.

This random sampling procedure made the research a lengthy process with considerable gaps between interviews. So although the random sampling was carried out by computer every month between August 1997 and July 1998, the 24 responses required from the BHTS users was only achieved by December 1998. Another factor which affected the length of the research was the stratification of the sample for ethnic minorities, who made up 50 per cent of the stratified sample (though only 20 per cent of the total number of home treatment users during

Table 4.1 Number of home treatment users sampled and number of interviews achieved

	Sampled		**Interviewed**	
	White	**Ethnic Minority**	**White**	**Ethnic Minority**
Male	6	6	5	5
Female	6	6	6	4
Total	12	12	11	9

this period). The reason for stratifying the sample in this way was because of our concern to fairly represent the views of a significant population living in the city of Bradford. There is still a lack of information on mental health issues within some ethnic minority communities and it is perceived locally – as well as nationally – that mental health services have yet to satisfactorily reach their needs (Fernando 1995; Henry 1999; Ramon 1996). Many ethnic minorities who suffer mental health problems in the Bradford area are economically disadvantaged and this was reflected in the larger number of this group who were not on the telephone and were sometimes in temporary accommodation. Consequently, it sometimes became rather like a game of 'cat and mouse' to locate these people and gain a response from them. Despite these factors, we achieved a high acceptance rate and reached our required 24 responses from the home treatment users (Table 4.1).

Twenty out of the 24 BHTS users sampled agreed to be interviewed. The positive response rate of 83 per cent – very high for any random sample – may reflect the author's closeness to the home treatment project, our determination to get a high acceptance rate or the high esteem in which many of the users held the BHTS.

4.3 The hospital sample

The hospital sample was made up of mental health users from all other sectors of Bradford apart from the BHTS sector of Ashgrove. This was done so that we could avoid the chance of accidentally interviewing a user who had previously received the BHTS or had experience of the different approach being undertaken in the Ashgrove sector. Unlike the home treatment sample, where the author had access to user names and addresses due to our own monitoring processes, with the hospital users the author had to liaise with the local psychiatric hospital's Information

Manager for access to names and addresses from the hospital database. Originally, we had decided that we would match the home treatment users interviewed as closely as possible with those who had received hospital treatment to be sure we were comparing like with like. Thus, a list of matching criteria was created which included diagnostic group, age group, gender, ethnic group, duration of admission, month of admission, and so on. If we had interviewed a white male 'schizophrenic' aged 16–24 who had been with home treatment for a period of two weeks and had been discharged in August 1997, for example, we would ask the Information Manager for a corresponding white male 'schizophrenic' who had been discharged from the hospital during the same month (seeing we were matching users and one user might refuse, we asked for preferably three people who matched the given criteria). These people would then be sent a letter similar to that for the home treatment users, asking for an interview (see Appendix A.3).

The initial problem was that the hospital database was not as extensive as our own research database. Some criteria we required were not recorded by the hospital, and the diagnostic category appeared on a separate database (the hospital was unsure as to how to link the two together). Another problem was that the hospital did not have enough people being discharged every month who matched such specific criteria. Further, the hospital was rather slow in dealing with such information requests, meaning that we usually had further people to match by the time the hospital information got back to us. Consequently, we received the first ten names and addresses (no telephone numbers, and most were ex-directory) towards the end of 1997. The information matched gender, ethnic group, age and month of discharge. The same letter was sent out to all of these people but the responses took a while to come back. The author eventually achieved two interviews from this sample of users.

Two issues became apparent from this experience. Firstly, the need for more names and addresses to each matched person to achieve a positive response and, secondly, the time delays involved in this process. Thus, the decision was taken to send out letters to *all* users discharged from hospital within a time period similar to that for home treatment users and, from the positive responses and interviews gained, to match retrospectively. So in May 1998 we sent out around 50 letters to hospital users, receiving positive responses from a further 11 users. The results of these sampling problems can be seen in Table 4.2.

The total number of hospital users interviewed was above what was required (29 compared to the 20 home treatment users interviewed),

Table 4.2 Number of hospital users sampled and number of interviews achieved

	Sampled		Interviewed	
	White	**Ethnic Minority**	**White**	**Ethnic Minority**
Male	5	5	13	2
Female	6	4	11	3
Total	11	9	24	5

though lower in terms of ethnic minority respondents (five as compared to nine interviews on the home treatment side), and therefore the overall sample is biased towards white groups and hospital users. For the majority of the hospital interviews we had to make our own assessment as to who was from an ethnic minority, so groups like the white Irish users (who are recorded as an ethnic minority for home treatment) are possibly in with the white users interviewed in the hospital group. What this means for the study is that the comparison of the home treatment and hospital user narratives could be biased towards the views of white hospital users. To lessen the impact of this, close attention was paid to ethnic minority views of hospital users (a kind of 'weighting' of minority narratives) as well as to ensuring that hospital users did not generally dominate the analysis simply because they were greater in number.

4.4 Piloting

A number of interviews were carried out with BHTS users in 1996 (see Cohen 1997a, 1997b) to assess the quality of service received, satisfaction with different features of the service, and user perceptions of distress and former psychiatric treatment. A pre-formalized questionnaire with a total of 60 open and closed questions was utilized. The questionnaire was changed several times as the interviews progressed with each lasting between one and two hours. What was particularly interesting and informative were the responses to the questions about psychiatry, the users' own understandings of their distress, as well as their ad hoc views – freely given – on their general life histories and experiences. These experiences often went beyond the subject of home treatment and psychiatric care. It was important to be able to explore these narratives further; there seemed to be important connections being made between psychiatry and a wider narrative involving life experience and change.

If this was meaningful expression of experience and thought for the users, why should it be ignored as irrelevant in making sense of one's life within the context of mental distress and recovery?

In studying mental illness, a number of pieces of research have looked at depression (Kleinman and Good 1985) and schizophrenia (Corin 1990; Fabrega 1989; Jenkins 1988; Lin and Kleinman 1988) within a general framework of cultural categories of knowledge and treatment, modified by individual experiences and circumstances (see Estroff *et al.* 1992). And there has been an expanding genre of first-person accounts (Murphy 1989; Zola 1982), as well as narrative analysis, of chronic illness experience (for example, Frank 1984; Kaufman 1988) which 'portray ingenious, exhaustive, and often ambivalent efforts to retain, redefine, even salvage a person from the engulfment of disabling illness' (Estroff *et al.* 1992: 337).

As we have seen in Chapter 2, narratives can take many different forms, including biography, autobiography, life history, diaries, journals and letters (Barbre and Personal Narratives Group 1989). In extracting user texts it was decided to allow users to speak on any matter they wanted to and for as long as they wanted to (there were no limits on this, people could talk about football for two hours if they so wished). A 'topic guide' was produced in case the narrative did not naturally 'flow' as expected. This topic guide could be used to trigger the narrative in cases where the conversation simply dried up. The method chosen for this research then, has a resemblance to 'open' (or 'informal') interviews. The research was exploratory in nature – the issues were for the mental health users to decide upon. The method allowed for a free-flowing narrative to be given by the mental health users with a minimum of preconceived issues being placed on the study. Given the lack of guidelines on 'writing as a scribe for the other' (see Denzin 1997: 231–49), the main idea of the method was to avoid direct questions, instead assisting the user in telling a life story or portraying some sort of narrative.

From the earlier interviews completed for the BHTS evaluation, a list of topics were drawn up (see Appendix A.4) and tested in a couple of pilot narrative interviews with previous users of the BHTS. A number of important discoveries were made from the pilots. One issue was that the topic guide was too specific in its approach and that the questions did not always appear to make sense to the user. For instance, the first pilot interview started,

> Q: 'So, what I'm interested in is, I wondered if you felt there were any crucial points in your life that either led to . . . first point of contact

with psychiatry, or maybe it was first points like where you've had real lows or real highs even?'

A: 'You want to know me first time I met psychiatrists?'

Q: 'Yeah.'

A: '(silence) Psychiatrists?'

Q: 'Yeah, but if there was points that like, where you were feeling down, you know, low about things.'

A: 'Well, I had been, wasn't exactly feeling low, well, I s'pose I must've been but about three or four years ago before I just went off it, were er, you know like when you know something's not quite right, you get a feeling then, you're not happy...' [user continues].

The user was quite laid-back in his approach to the interview but still found the researcher's initial mentioning of periods of 'highs' and 'lows' (as mentioned in the work of Gergen 1994) disconcerting, eventually relating this back to his first contact with psychiatrists and then embarking on a narrative of what led up to this first encounter with psychiatry. This caused the author to revise the topic guide to broader issues (see Appendix A.5). Often the topic guide was only used when people gave minimal responses. The length and composition of the narrative was going to vary considerably as one might expect. In the case of the pilots, the first narrative was half an hour, the second narrative over two hours. In the author's view, the first made sense but the second came across, initially, as an eclectic and erratic worldview which was difficult to understand or place. One passage extracted from this text is shown below:

> Thing is, as a kid I was always sort of pressurised to do things, you just tend to rebel, you don't want to do. You get to the stage where you just want to get on with things and erm, you can't. And you start blaming the environment, or people around you, you know, not being understanding or whatever. You know deep down inside that the only person who can do anything about it is yourself, you've just got to motivate yourself, shut yourself away from the rest of the world and not pay any attention to what they must think or make of it. You've got to find ways of making it interesting and making it work. Now, like I say, you've got to break up that monotony by doing other things. I could never organise myself, you know, to do sort of other things and keep my music side going at the same time. I'd hit on something. For me it would mean a total break in my music and that's how I've always gone about things, the wrong way. Now

you know I'd be happy if I was to erm, get some kind of order and discipline in my life, get up at 9 am and then enjoy full day... say every day of the week, for 52 weeks of the year. That would be great. I found that at one point, I'd got into a rut. I wouldn't be getting out of bed until 2 pm and my day would be squandered and that was a short outbearing [?] really, weren't able to, able to go out then really. Basically, you just hibernate, you know, which to me spelt danger, you know what I mean? Just got more and more withdrawn, more and more worried and het-up about everything, and I don't think there was anybody around to help at the time. Our kid would come round, lazy sod (laughs), sleeping all day, he don't do anything, he don't want to hear it, you know what you're doing, you're just looking for, erm you know, a way out, you know, and erm, as I say, there was no one around and you give up on a lot of things. It'd have done me well at the time to speak to a psychiatrist, I think it'd have been handier if I'd have had a shrink at school, you know what I mean? (laughs). So, back at school, I was a bit of a megalomaniac (laughs). Old guitar, I'll find it, you know. Everyone, sort of... estimates of potential, could do anything, or achieve anything you set out to do with life and, er, you realise where it gone... nothing's ever straight-cut and er... wrecked. Now I'm sort of banking on a job you know, I need to clean-up now and get myself smart and get, er... I need to feel good about myself, I suppose in the way I dress, like I say, things'll put themselves right as time progresses. You know, I've started getting back into my books and that, er, I went through a period when I used to get books out of the library and need... basically. Read the headings on each chapter, maybe read a full book, just draw my own conclusions, shut the book and never pick up the book again. I'm saying, got to a stage now where you know if I do pick up a book, I'll read it all the way through and I make sure I've grasped the whole story like and not just drawn my own conclusions. I suppose I've just been living in my own fantasy world, you know, you see so much on television and you think, oh yeah, it's just the same thing, you know, happening all over, erm, but it ain't. It's like erm, well I don't really want to go on about books that I've read, erm, there's so much you can learn books that I've read, erm, there's so much you can learn about character (silence)... There's nowt to prove reading a book whereas, you know, on television a lot of these, sort of... a lot of articles and that portray... it is just totally discarded you know, you can just get on with the action, it doesn't really explain the individual as a whole. Erm, no, like I say, I believe that, you know, it's going to help me as

> an individual and I promise, I promise to do more reading, erm, I'm not very good at, erm, socialising, mingling would do.

When I read this passage again more than a year later – after completing nearly 50 narrative interviews – it seemed quite a structured and thought-out passage, with the user giving an account of his life history which includes his childhood, his passions, his feelings of being separated from the world but also being part of that world and his determination to 'do better' in the future. Yet the author's own confusion and insecurities in how to 'understand' the sheer variety in such narratives at the time made this life story seem quite fractured and displaced. At this point in the research process it was necessary to reaffirm that this study was about representing mental health user beliefs, perceptions and realties, rather than the author's. Fundamentally, each narrative carries equal worth.

4.5 Narrative collection

Interviews were carried out in the users' homes unless they wished them to be done elsewhere. When this was the case, they usually preferred to be interviewed at the author's office at the University of Bradford. In the case of some users – who could be either BHTS or hospital-only users – who had been re-hospitalized, the interviews were carried out there. The time and date for interview was left in the hands of the users, with some interviews being carried out mid-evening or on a weekend. At the interview it was explained that we were interested in their experiences of psychiatry and more generally their life experiences, and that the interview was confidential and anonymous. We wished the users to feel that the interview was in their hands and that they could tell us anything they wanted to, and if there were questions that came up that they did not want to answer they could move on to other topics. Finally, it was stated that we would like to tape the interview to get an accurate record of the conversation but if they were unhappy with this, we could take notes with pen and paper. It was emphasized that, if recorded, the tapes would be typed-up and then destroyed; only the researcher and the transcriber would have access to the tapes in the meantime.

Ten of the 49 users interviewed preferred not to be taped. This obviously affected the quality of the narratives collected and, more importantly, is another step removed from the reporting of a personal narrative. It can be argued that the transcription from a tape gives a much more accurate 'interpretation' of the narrative than a researcher's notes of that narrative. The users were usually alone when they were interviewed, but in a number of cases a friend or family member would be in the background, which could in turn have an effect on the narrative given to us. In the case of our bilingual researcher (who was trained with the topic guide and given extensive background on narrative approaches), when she interviewed ethnic minority users it was necessary for her – as a Muslim woman – not to be alone in a room with a man. In these cases – after seeking agreement from the user – she would attend the interview with her young daughter. Again, this may have affected the narrative conversation received.

Users were aware that the bilingual researcher and the author were both from the University of Bradford and that we were interested in their experiences of psychiatry. Given the background to these interviews, the usual place to start was by asking them about their first experience of psychiatry. This led to an array of issues which either the users followed through themselves or could be followed up by further queries on their thoughts, feelings, life events, work and other aspects which fell outside of their experiences of the psychiatric system. The way users dealt with this narrative style of interview can be roughly divided into three responses: firstly, the proactive users who were only too happy to talk without much, if any, prompting from the researcher; secondly, the static one-word responses which led to much prompting but still very short interviews; and, thirdly, users who were more comfortable with a standard question and answer format at first, but then would return to expand more on earlier themes later in the interview. The following user, for example, needed only one word from the interviewer to initiate a response:

Q: 'Right.'

A: 'Right then, I'm gonna read a poem and it's entitled "My son", that's [Joseph]. Well, it's not a poem it's, it's a bit of a caption really, you know what a caption is don't you? It's, it's saying words and they're all put together... by, well by me, so here... goes. "My dear sons and daughters" – title – he's just about to [be] born now and I can hear them crying and it starts, "crying in the theatre of life, now my darling children, now my darling child or children, you're with us well to the drama of life you've been called from your sleep to awaken, our babies from afar, how you have traveled...".' [user continues]

With this narrative we are already discovering personal details and it has not been necessary to introduce any subjects or topics to the user.

However, the opposite could happen in other cases, where we would have to start by asking quite direct questions and then hope the user would illuminate further without additional probing. The following start of an interview highlights this difficulty:

Q: 'I mean, I mean generally there are, the service you received, were you happy?'
A: 'Yeah.'
Q: 'Yeah, alright then?'
A: 'Yes, everything was alright.'
Q: 'Anything particularly good about it?'
A: '[People?] in general was alright.'
Q: 'Yeah?'
A: 'Yeah... I don't know, it was alright. Everything alright.'
Q: 'They help you out ok?'
A: 'Yeah. Made me feel better, yeah.'
Q: 'Was it... is that your first period of like... psychiatric treatment?'
A: 'Mm. Yeah.'
Q: 'Alright.'
A: 'Yeah.'
[interview continues]

A number of interviews were similar, with the answers remaining quite uniform despite continued probing and leaving long pauses in case further information was forthcoming. It was evident that this 'narrative approach' may not work equally successfully with everyone; there is the automatic response to an interaction with a researcher which suggests that he or she will have a list of questions to which responses can then be given. There is an assumed set of procedures when one meets for an interview, and to try to alter this interaction – as was done in this study – can upset the balance. Nevertheless, we should not reject the responses of any of the users as simply 'bad responses' or 'bad interviews'. These are their statements and their realities and it is important for us to assess them as such, rather than suggesting that they obviously had much more to say that they were unwilling to share with us.

4.6 Narrative analysis

The average length of the narrative conversation was one and a half hours, with the resulting 49 interviews producing a total of around 500 pages of text. The analysis of these narratives is central to the study, not only in terms of demonstrating the effectiveness of a new 'method' of research but also in understanding the lives of those who have experienced psychiatric hospital or home treatment.

Although software packages are available for the analysis of qualitative information, these are counterproductive to an interpretative ethnographic view of 'acting as a scribe for the other' and accurately recording personal narratives. Software, such as N6 (formerly known as 'NUD.IST'), facilitates 'cutting and pasting' exercises which subtract parts of individual texts and places them into different categories created by the researcher for generalizability of the 'text data'. It remains my belief that, for any form of qualitative analysis, there is no substitute to reading and re-reading hard copies of the texts (granted, this can also be done with a PC as well!). The texts must be taken in their entirety before any further analysis is considered. Naturally, this was significant in presenting the user narratives outlined in the following chapter. The user narratives had to remain as closed to the original texts as possible, allowing for the practicality of book space (see Chapter 5). However, a second part of the analysis drew on all the narratives and required more traditional methods of investigation. This time, the text was 'cut and pasted' into different categories (such as 'social and economic factors' and 'self-coping techniques') using N6. The text from each category was then printed out in hard copy. The hard copies were then read through again and brief notes were made of the main points in the text, the notes were then copied onto paper and similar points were put together (for instance within the 'meaning of illness' category, a number of 'hearing voices' experiences would be put together). A number of tables were produced and commented on, and portions of the text were reproduced where appropriate (see Chapters 6 and 7).

As a result, the analysis is presented not as a construction of a life within psychiatry but rather a construction of the place of psychiatry, mental health and other factors within a life. Though it is true that some users had experienced psychiatry on and off for many years and felt it was a significant part of their lives, others had had one or two experiences and saw these periods as less significant within their narrative. For these reasons, the analysis chapters in this book are structured in the following way: Chapter 5 investigates a sample of the narratives produced in terms of textuality, consistency, fluidity, plurality and meaning. Chapters 6 and 7 look at the main issues which were highlighted from the analysis of all the narratives, namely, people's life histories, psychiatric experiences, social and economic lives, personal experiences of illness, self-coping and future activities, with comparisons between home treatment and hospital narratives being made wherever possible. Chapter 6 focuses on the descent into illness and experiences of psychiatry, whereas Chapter 7 looks at issues of recovery and self-coping. The analysis attempts to capture the essence of the personal narratives by demonstrating structural curiosities, speech and symbols, and what these might mean within a context of 'illness' constructions. Though it has not been possible to reproduce all the narrative texts within this book, it conveys both an analysis of general trends – where they are found to exist – and the primacy of the individual text.

4.7 Conclusion

This chapter has summarized the practical implications of taking a narrative approach within health research. We have also considered the difficulties of introducing a new 'methodology', and the problems of collection and analysis of the resulting information. The proof of the success of this research lies within the rich quality of the resulting texts. In Chapters 5–7 the user narratives are outlined, shedding new light on the lives of people who, for whatever reason, have experienced psychiatric treatment.

5
The User Narratives

> Last night, I just ended up... playing my old singles. Just to remember what it was like to be young again and stuff like that. So I'm playing all my David Bowie singles and stuff, and 'Transformer' and Lou Reed and all.
>
> (Anne)

5.1 Summary

In the previous chapters I have outlined the theoretical background as well as the methodological considerations to the research in this book. This chapter outlines eight narratives from mental health users: four who experienced the Bradford Home Treatment Service and four who experienced hospital treatment only. This is done to attempt comparison of the narratives. Further, the four users in each group represent male and female users and white and minority groups equally (that is, one white female, one white male, one minority female and one minority male), so the gender and ethnicity of users within each group are fairly represented here. Denzin (1997: 225) has stated,

> The reflexive, epiphanic, messy text redefines the ethnographic project. The writer-as-scribe for the other also becomes a cultural critic: a person who voices interpretations about the events recorded and observed. At the same time, as the scribe of a messy text the writer shapes the poetic narrative representations that are brought to the people studied.

Consequently, the research work is a testing ground on which social science is 'remade' through new ethnographic approaches.

The four home treatment narratives and the four hospital narratives were chosen from, respectively, the 20 and 29 user narratives collected for each group during the fieldwork. They have not been chosen randomly but rather on the basis of the amount of information gleaned from the users themselves. If the narrative had a 'flow' to it and was seen to follow the user's account of his or her story (rather than the interviewer's story) it was considered to be more relevant to include this narrative as a 'good example' of a user narrative. The selection is thus highly subjective and it is for this reason that further analysis is carried out on all the narratives in Chapters 6 and 7. It is not the case that the narratives presented in this chapter particularly 'make more sense' than other narratives; rather they represent a cross section of narratives which allows the reader to contemplate new and alternative 'readings' of the accounts of psychiatric users compared to those that have appeared in previous studies.

At the same time, the narratives illustrated here use the author's own understanding of the main points of the user texts. As it is not possible to detail the total narrative within this chapter – this would have used up at least half of the total space for the book – I have selected the portions of text that would seem of most relevance to the user as his or her story progresses. Occasionally the author has summarized background histories, current opinions and so on, to keep the text to a manageable size. The author has also summarized and contextualized parts of the narrative as it progresses, whilst simultaneously attempting to avoid any direct interpretation or deconstruction of the texts. As a result, what appears in this chapter is by and large maintenance of the user's own accounts of their lives, rather than the author's narrative of user narratives.

With these issues in mind, what has been achieved is a fair and accurate account of psychiatric user narratives. The author has attempted to place himself within the narratives and to be honest about the background to the production of these texts rather than ignore the place of the researcher vis-à-vis the interviewee. For the reason of accuracy of each narrative, 'corrections' to the texts presented have been avoided. Some of the text may not appear to make literal 'sense' in the form in which it appears. Given these texts were transcribed by a third party (and two of the narratives were translated by our bilingual researcher), it is possible that these are mistakes or errors of others rather than that of the 'direct narrative' from the mouths of the users. We cannot be sure of this, however, so the texts have been left as they appeared on being returned from the transcribers. The only exceptions to this was when a word had been obviously spelt wrong in the transcribed text and was corrected by the author, the insertion of an explanation to the passage by the author with '[brackets]', or the anonymizing of names and replacement with a description such as '[husband]'. The transcribers have used (brackets) for particular noises on the tapes, or used '[?]' when the transcriber has been unsure of a particular word (this is particularly the case with the names of medications). The transcribers have also signified when the recording was inaudible with three full stops (. . .). Pseudonyms have been used instead of real names for the users and any information that appeared in the text that could possibly reveal the user's identity to a third party has been hidden. When a conversation between the researcher and the user is cited, this is noted by 'Q' (researcher) and 'A' (user) before the relevant text. In line with attempting to write more in a literary style (see Denzin 1997), the author uses the first-person 'I' within this chapter (instead of using terms such as 'the author', 'the researcher' or 'we') and adds some brief anecdotal introductions to the text where relevant. Following the eight narratives, I will summarize some comparative aspects of the user narratives before briefly considering the wider issues that emerge from the presented texts.

Finally, a note for those readers who may not be accustomed to the Yorkshire dialect. Those across the Atlantic may be most familiar with the dialect from television series such as 'All Creatures Great and Small' or 'Last of the Summer Wine'; more recent films such as 'Brassed Off' or 'The Full Monty' have presented the accent to a wider audience. The narratives occasionally illustrate the use of this dialect, for instance, in the abbreviation of words such as 'isn't it' ('innit'), 'doesn't it' ('dunnit'), 'them' ('em') and 'nothing' ('nowt'). Another commonality in the dialect is to shorten the words 'to' or 'the' to 't', such as in 't'finish' (to finish), 't'doctors' (the doctors), 't'treatment' (the treatment) and so on. Although I lived and worked in Bradford for six years, as a 'Southerner' I cannot claim an expert knowledge on the wonderful eccentricities of the Yorkshire people (for more on the Yorkshire dialect including a glossary of terms, see BBC 2005).

5.2 Hospital narrative: Philip

It is early evening but already dark. I am on the edge of a Bradford housing estate and I am cold and wet. I find the right house at the second attempt. Philip greets me at the door with a friendly smile. He asks if it is alright for his mum and grandma to be in the room whilst we do the interview. No problem with me if it is no problem with him. After getting me some tea, we sit down at one side of his cosy front room and after the usual assurances (of confidentiality and so forth) we are into the narrative:

> Right, well from the first day that I became ill I went to my GP [General Practitioner]. It started on the shop floor at a firm called [firm name] and... I thought I were persecuted at work. Definitely you know, people walking past, making little remarks and then just sodding off without resolving anything and they just kept, you know, a lot of people all on the shop floor working as a electrical fitter and there are about two hundred people. A lot of contractors on the shop floor, so it were in a really highly charged atmosphere, you see, and it started there.

The relevance of the firm being an electronics company becomes clear later in Philip's narrative. His comment that it was a 'highly charged atmosphere' could be seen as a useful metaphor for much of the narrative that follows. He continues,

> Anyway, I'd been there about a year at this place. So I went to the manager and I told him that I were being persecuted by a certain group of people on the shop floor and he just said 'go and see your doctor'. So he wasn't prepared to do anything about it. So what happened was, I blacked out on the shop floor and I was standing by a panel. I were panel wiring and I was standing by this panel and I blacked out and in front of me. You know, inside the front of my head just went blank inside. Total black out and when I looked again, I didn't collapse or anything, I was still stood. I looked at the clock and I'd lost an hour. So anyway eventually the, the sort of persecution got too much and eventually I were like a sort of dog, a dog chasing its tail. So I finished there anyway.

There are plenty of theories to explain what Philip was going through: the social pressures of the working environment he encountered leading to a breakdown, physiological problems leading to the blackouts, psychological problems of isolation from his peer group leading to paranoid feelings and so on. After visiting the psychiatrist he is told he is paranoid, taken into hospital and medicated with Promazine, a major tranquilizer. Philip tells me he cried when he was first diagnosed: 'it was something I fear, that I had a great amount of fear about being "mad" in inverted commas. I didn't want to be mad. I didn't want to be put away'. Prescribed to relive anxiety, taking the medication led to a 'deep, deep depression'. He persuaded the doctors to change his medication. Like many users I interviewed, he was still on psychotropic medication yet very negative about it. At one point he says,

> Psychotic drugs really are bad. I mean I've just tried Risperdal [an antipsychotic medication] which is the latest thing. It's supposed to be up to and it cut, it cut me sex system off altogether. So if I masturbated, it were just a dry one, completely dry. So that sort of thing and everything went co, it's like it were freezing me. It was cooling me down inside and lots of other things that, small things like you get, you get, it's like somebody's controlling you.

And control would appear to be Philip's central problem. He comments on his current medication, Sulpiride, another antipsychotic drug:

> The Sulpiride's not perfect, but it's better than Clozapine [another antipsychotic medication] and it's better than Risperdal, but it still, it doesn't remove the voices you know, and the source of the voices is the source of the conspiracy against me. So what I've got to do is find out who's, 'cos all it is, is somebody in my head and 'you are', 'you do', 'you know'. It's that part of language that never intermates anything, but you do. It's telling you that 'you do', 'you are', 'you know', 'you will'. So when you're the thought you'll just respond to it all the time. It's like somebody's sat behind me on a computer with a mouth piece, reading it off the wire.

Philip feels controlled by others through the voices in his head that are conspiring against him. He tells me the talking in his head can be so loud that he cannot concentrate on the studies he would like to continue in the future. At the same time he is taking psychotropic medication to try and 'control' (or remove) the voices. But Philip's conspirators also have the technology and the means by which to take his thoughts from him and broadcast them to others. In fact, the emphasis in Philip's narrative is on surveillance and the transmission of these conspiratorial messages to him and from him through all means of electrical gadgetry. As Philip explained to me of the illness,

> This is to do with somebody transmitting signals to my brain and also receiving. I mean I've been on the television. They eavesdrop on the television. If you look, what happens is, you look at the telly from the ... 'Question Time' [television show]. I'm looking at the television, all of a sudden round the table with Jonathan Dimbleby [television broadcaster] or whoever it is, David Dimbleby [television broadcaster] sorry. Yeah, there's John Edwards [famous artist] the first one. So there's David Dimbleby, then John Edwards there and all of a sudden there's a pause. Right and a 'bigger', the word 'bigger' flies out of my head and into the studio, right, and it just goes behind 'em, so they can hear me saying 'bigger' and John Redwood [Member of Parliament] says 'well we know what happens to them don't we?' So it's that sort of thing. On 'Shooting Stars' [television show], I've been on 'Shooting Stars', in the back, and all of a sudden they're all looking at and then you just see their eye balls go up a little bit and they're listening, 'cos it's behind. The sound comes in behind, so the sound man's doing it. So he flicks the sound in and whatever it is, some irrational nonsense that came out of my head at the time. So not only are they eavesdropping, but they're stealing my thought. Which you know, is an original thought. No matter how stu, I mean a lot of its crap but I'll give you that. A lot of its complete crap but there are, there are original ideas in there that shouldn't be taken out.

This broadcasting of Philip's thoughts is an invasion of his privacy, even if what is transmitted is trivial why should everyone who has access to such technology have access to his own thoughts? Sometimes what is transmitted from his thoughts can be more distressing. He mentions listening to 'Talk Radio', a national radio show hosted by the journalist Peter Deeley, of whom Philip says,

> It's like he's sat, he's got his computer and he's got everything and he can read off the wire what's happening inside my head whilst he's taking a call, or he can hear something in his phones or something like that and then he can fuse them and fuse across. And one night I was listening to Peter Deeley and there was this girl on the line. She was just wingeing about something, she were in distress and all of a sudden I got this feeling in my head and it just went 'slag'. Like that and then I heard it on the radio 'slag' and then I heard the girl cry and then the phone went dead.

Philip comments on this episode,

> What had happened was Peter Deeley had crossed over. So it's like a double cross. So the moment he came out he, or the engineer did. It's an engineering thing innit? The engineer crossed it over and picked it out at her end, so she got it. Now I, I can't affect that. If somebody starts taking thought out my head, the bad stuff, and sequencing it like that through a satellite system or whatever. It's amazing, it's just biological weapons. It can take my thought and you can give it to every television company in the world. They can do what they like. So I could walk up to Gerry Adams [Northern Ireland politician] tomorrow, 'this is what... thinks of you'. You know, its weird innit? But it's right.

Given this narrative, it is not surprising that Philip was affronted when his psychiatrist asked him personal questions about living at home with his mother and so forth. This was not the issue for Philip. He freely admits that 'the only thing I get out of [the psychiatrist] is a certificate with a drug on it'. There is a 'logic' to Philip's narrative, but it conflicts with psychiatry's narrative. No room is given to Philip's personal construction of reality. Therefore, when speaking with his psychiatrist about his illness and asking, 'what would you do then? What would you do?', the psychiatrist actually got angry with him. Philip calls his psychiatric records 'the most bungled piece of literature I've ever noticed in my life'. Included within the records are police reports from a forensic psychiatrist who Philip had spoken to following a car accident. Although the conversation was taped, Philip maintains that the psychiatrist lied in the resulting report which, among other things, suggested that Philip's mother had had an affair (Philip's mother interrupts at this point to agree with the narration). Philip now feels many of these professionals are also a part of the conspiracy against him.

Through the narrative, however, Philip is not denying the fact that he has a problem or an illness, he even uses a psychiatric diagnosis himself ('schizophrenia'), but he also feels that psychiatry is of little use in helping him get 'better'. The reason why he initially saw the forensic psychiatrist was that he thought that the car accident may have had something to do with his illness. Both Philip and his mother wonder if I myself might have any suggestions at the end of the interview. I believe this is what psychiatrists call 'insight'; it is acknowledgement by the person that they have an illness and that they need to seek help for it, yet psychiatry seems incapable of doing their bit and making him well again. Perhaps 'well again' is not a possibility for Philip. He sums his problem up by acknowledging,

> *A*: 'There's no way I could prove any of this and I wouldn't go by your psychiatric records, but if I wanted to take, say, what I want ideally is a lawyer who believes in me and who'll defend me. So I can get them to stop. I mean they're not there now, but I'm talking to you, but as soon as you've gone you know, they'll start again "thought you were believable didn't you, big virgin bastard?" Like that, you know, and it just gets worse and worse all the time. It's a pain in the arse. I haven't committed a crime, that's the thing. I were working on that shop floor and I did what my gaffa. I got on well with my gaffa and suddenly they all conspired to do me and the reason is virginity.'
>
> *Q*: 'Virginity?'
>
> *A*: 'Yeah, mine is, 'cos they were sort of picking holes in me all the time. You know they decided I was, so fair enough. Just the way I work I think. I always draw that, that reaction, you know. There's nothing I can do about it.'

So in a few sentences Philip has summed up the problem he is having, why he has the problem and how he might deal with it. Philip loved the work and he describes his workmates as a very intelligent group of people, though he sometimes felt apart from them and this eventually led to them starting to persecute him. He explains,

> Well they're engineers, they can needle [?] everything they can use. Well that, that's the way I see it anyway. I could walk up that street and just about every house that's got an alarm can send a signal, or I can receive a signal from it and it can send one to me and it's all in the sequential logic of everything. So if they, if they got the finger on the pulse. If they can send a signal from the control room, down through the system to a particular house. To a particular television. To a particular electrode. To a transmitter. To the smallest instrumentation in that box there, through the sound and also the decoder. They can affect the coding that's being transmitted to the aerial and they can get in there, underneath it or above it or whatever, but they'll get into it anyway, because all the time we're listening to the radio. We're coming through and it merges. So you start with, you start with [work colleagues names] in a cycle. They're the ones that are giving me the jip. They're the worlds nerds [?]. Then you've got

> another group of people who are on the top shelf, radio presenters and television presenters. So you merge these two together and then they on the radio on the end can hear exactly what I'm thinking as well. So they've joined in. The conspiracy is massive.

Given the size of the conspiracy against Philip one might expect him to be very upset and depressed, whereas he appears – at least for the duration of the interview – rather positive about his illness and the conspiracy. Maybe this is partly because the conspirators have the power to make Philip feel very good as well. As he explains, the conspirators,

> Make it better 'cos they're controlling it. When I seriously good quality times, they give me the feeling in the head. The feeling through the body sometimes. I mean feeling simple, it's just, it's just like I'm talking about chemicals now. I'm talking about feelings just. I've very little to do with thought anyway. More to do with just the way you feel. So they can make me feel good if they want or they can make me feel bad. So if they're pumping, when they started, they were pumping energy into me at an enormous rate and I was just sort of, my brain were bursting out of my head. It was the same thing all the time – 'thought you were unbelievable, didn't you, big bastard?' But they use a phonetics as well, it's not just 'big bastard' all the time, its 'big baaastard, big baaastard', like that, screaming and shouting. It's like somebody slating you for a complete century, you know. It just goes on and on and on, and you wonder why you're being bollocked and you just don't know why.

He admits 'there are funny bits to it [the illness], but it's basically stealing original material I think'. I ask him if he's tried anything apart from the drugs that have lessened the voices or made him feel better, and I'm rather surprised by the answer he gives. 'The first thing I did when I became ill', Philip replies,

> I started cycling and I thought there were some sort of physiological process at work and if I cycled and exercised I'd get a release, a breakdown, the nasty chemicals that are supposed to decode me, but then it were technical, like a technical thing. I were being told by the psychiatrist that it were me, it were in me you know. I sort of define it myself although they led me to believe that I was some sort of weirdo... but I don't, but I know I used to cycle. I cycled for four hours with me mates. We went on this cycle ride. When I came back

> I was clear as a bell, but I can't cycle for four hours a day and that's all. If I cycled for four hours every day I'd be fit as a fiddle and the voices would just go, 'cos they wouldn't be there, but I'd have to go out every day come rain or shine and cycle four hours a day. That would keep it at bay altogether.

I am a little astonished at this revelation, which seems rather matter-of-fact to Philip. Maybe there is not a 'cure', but he has just outlined a way of ridding himself of these voices which would appear to be what he wants to do (as well as find the conspirators). But maybe this is because of my own focus on the illness which he has outlined in some detail over the past hour. Maybe his life is not as centred on the illness as I had thought? Maybe just proving to himself that he is not the 'weirdo' is enough? For when it comes to it, Philip seems concerned to do other things rather than four hours of cycling a day, even if it is only smoking, drinking tea and listening to the radio or watching television. He also has a number of friends who he visits. He sometimes plays guitar. Though he denies it, his mother tells me Philip has done a lot of studying over the years. Nevertheless, he admits,

> I'm going to do a degree. I'm just telling them [the voices] that as soon as you piss off I'll start studying and do something and make something of myself or whatever, and until you piss off I'm not doing anything. I've sorted taken two years out [from university] now and I only intended to take a year out, but I had a massive trauma in Manningham [a district in the centre of Bradford], so... so I haven't studied. So I should go back. I'm going to sign up for university after Christmas for definite this year. I've said I'm gonna do it and I'm gonna do it.

So despite the conspirators and the voices, there seems to be a definite future objective for Philip. Maybe this is his way of taking control of his life and overcoming his illness? On my exit he leaves me with one last statement: 'I'll sum it up by saying it's definitely dungeons and dragons'.

5.3 Home treatment narrative: Michael

Verging on the countryside, a few miles out of the city centre of Bradford, I find Michael's stone cottage. A cigarette and a mug of tea, then I ask him if he feels anything in particular led to the point of his crisis:

> My marriage break-up, really it were that led to me to be into depression. I've had a difficult life all my life, and I suppose I've had depression on and off throughout my life really, but my marriage break-up were my last straw really. It just sort of broke me mentally, as it tends to do.

Michael is 32, divorced and has three children; he is self-employed and often works away from home. These factors appear to be central to his illness narrative, 'it's taken its toll on me a bit really,' he tells me. Marriage, particularly had 'deeply instilled a lot of insecurity in me,' he comments, and even with subsequent relationships he relates back to his problems with the marriage. However, Michael is keen to stress the help given by the BHTS with his situation and this becomes a constant theme of the narrative. For instance, he remarks,

> I was in quite a bad state of distress actually, when I met them [BHTS] and they did come out and help me a lot, a lot of in-depth talking, in-depth work, and they've gone out of their way as well to help me in other areas, which really aren't their department I suppose. Like getting access to my children and stuff like that, they've helped me out in a lot of areas, so they do go out of their way to help you in any respect really.

Michael's narrative also contains many comments about the way he has been in the past and how he has been helped by psychiatry, especially the BHTS, to a better position now. He continues to see himself needing long-term help, particularly counselling. He mentions at one juncture, 'I have had clinical depression you see, which is quite a severe depression and when I am depressed, I'm depressed and there's no way out of it for me, it's just a downward spiral'. As well as BHTS – who have offered him the time and space to talk through his problems – hospital has also been welcomed as a 'break' from his troubles. I ask him if he does anything himself that helps him feel better,

> Yeah, I think it's just positive thinking really, in't it? I tend to, I'm a bit of a negative person really, I tend to think on the worst side and then I don't get any unexpected hiccups, its... but just getting out actually, just getting out and about which is what I'd actually stopped doing, I'd stopped going out, I'd stopped working, I'd stopped looking for work and I just turned everything into negatives all the time. And I suppose you've got to get a... positive thoughts there at times

> haven't you, in order to get on with your life. And I think they [BHTS] helped me to do that, keep looking, keep thinking positive and things will change eventually, and I suppose they have really.

It is maybe a straightforward narrative of illness. Michael has lost contact with much of his family and old friends. He admits it was always the way, from childhood onwards, to walk away from situations if he had disagreements with people. At the same time he has found it difficult not having these people around him anymore. It has been the same in relationships, though he says now, 'I'm finding a bit more strength in staying, really, and working out a relationship'. Though he does not like the vulnerability involved in having to stay and work things out, he realizes it is necessary if he wants a relationship to develop. Michael is now going through the legal system to gain access to his children and is positive that it is the right course of action, rather than trying to sort these issues out himself, which used to significantly add to his depression.

Michael also mentions that the friends he used to go out with would usually end up in trouble and fights, which he became wary of after a while. He felt he had outgrown the group and wanted to create a 'new', 'better' life for himself. He says of these times,

> Yeah, well it were constantly, week after week, and needless trouble, 90 percent of it, just needless. But they'd [his friends] be thinking it were funny and having a good laugh about it, and they'd meet up next day and 'oh, wasn't that a good night last night?', and to me it wasn't a good night at all and it never would be a good night but they seemed to find the humor in it. As I say, I'd known 'em from, well, 15 years, a lot of them friends. and I suppose when I met them that's actually what I were like – I'd just left home and just come out of all that trouble with all the, all the misgivings, and I'd carried it over and I were a bit of a violent person to be honest, I were aggressive and outgoing but now I see myself, I've quietened, I'm quite a staid [?] person now really, like I've toned down a lot of me faults, a lot of me faults.

This narrative illustrates that there is no natural course into or out of illness. There is no easy way through the illness for Michael, interacting with people is bound to involve emotional input and the result is not always positive. Michael is quite positive about all the treatment he received, whether through the BHTS's one-to-one help or the hospital's care for him. He feels the anti-depressive medication also helps him. He was able to relax when he was at hospital, though he also feels he received more intensive counselling and input from the BHTS. He also has sessions with a psychologist, which opens some of the old wounds and leaves him upset and emotional. Nevertheless, Michael feels the therapy is necessary, trusting the professionals he deals with:

> Yeah, it's very upsetting as I say, a lot of things that are in my life, that have happened in my life, are very deep painful things, so it is upsetting to me when I go, but I've been going through this now for so long that I can virtually talk to anybody about the deep problems that I feel and the things that hurt me, and I'm quite free to air my views on everything, to anybody really. So there is that trust there that it is all private and confidential.

Michael may be becoming the expert on his own problems. He admits to being too confused to be able to deal with his problems in the past, but due to the BHTS's input he now feels that he can 'sit down in clarity and sort my problems out'. He still envisages needing a few years of counselling given 'things are that deep' but he can now see 'a light at the end of the tunnel'. Previously, he felt that he was going 'round and round in circles' all his life, but now he sees 'a bit of a straight road'. I ask him if there was anything positive to come out of his illness. He replies,

> I think I've learned to relax a bit more about problems and see that everybody has problems, it's not just me with my problems, so I do feel a bit clearer in my thinking. Yeah, definitely more relaxed in my approach to problems and the way I want my life to be. The person I think I am, I feel I understand myself a lot better now. Now that I've related the person I am now is just a by-product of my childhood if you like, and we're all products of other people's making to some extent, aren't we? And I suppose that's what, I can look at myself now and see the person I am and why I am the person I am, and take steps to change what I don't like about myself. So I do have a better understanding of myself as a result of all this. So that's one good thing I suppose.

5.4 Hospital narrative: Rachel

For once, I have a car to get to the interview, which is just as well as it is raining again and I am on a sprawling housing estate on the edge of Bradford, populated with a number of different-sized blocks of flats as well as terraced housing. I find the right block without much trouble but end up wandering all the way around it looking for the (almost concealed) door to get inside. When I see the security man on duty I ask him for directions to the appropriate floor, after confirming who I am seeing and where I have to go he mutters 'you've picked a right time to visit'. I ask him what he means by this and receive the reply, 'you'll see'. Rather ominous. This is not the sort of thing I like to hear and my brain starts working overtime as to what to do if this turns into the hypothetical *bad research situation* which I have yet to experience in my many years in the job. It is for this reason that I am somewhat surprised when a very jolly woman greets me at the front door. We sit down with coffee and I am immediately told, 'well I don't know what happened to me, I was just deranged, I was, you know, stood out in the middle of the road trying to get knocked down'. 'Really?', I respond. She continues:

> I had these voices in my head telling me that I've, this is what I've got to do. Anyhow, I think as it happened nobody'd knock me down, but I went over to the vicar's and I spent the night in the vicarage, and he knew that there was something not right about, well it were obvious I wasn't right, so they just put me up there [in the psychiatric hospital].

What emerges from Rachel is a fascinating illness narrative (this is witnessed by my repeated 'oh, goshs' on the interview tape). She experienced two years of illness, but now it is gone and she is getting on with her life. This is how she explains it:

> The first time, it was two years, it was when, the first year that he [her son] went away to university, and they [the psychiatrists] said it's 'cos he's gone away, but I never thought that it was, because, you know, he hasn't always been with me – he's lived with his dad, you know what I mean, and we've moved about and that, and it weren't, I don't think that it was that. In my own mind now after all this time I think, 'cos of what these voices were telling me, they were trying to tell me that I'd got an illness, you know, I were seriously ill and I had cancer...And I kept going through this, they were just nightmares of going to my own funeral and horrible things that kept going on in my head, you know, and I couldn't sort it out, and after two years that's what they diagnosed was matter with me: I had breast cancer.

> ...And when I came round [in hospital], it were just like I used to come round when I were in [the psychiatric hospital], with all these drips on me and, you know, tubes coming out of me, and that's what happened to me.... It frightened me 'cos it were all, you know, when I went, when I was there laid in t'coffin in this, 'cos you know like there's curtains round your bed.... And I was laid there with these curtains round my bed and I, to me I was just laid in a coffin and I could see the, the funeral flowers and I, I just kept thinking that I was dead. It was horrendous.
>
> ...Then last year when they found that I had got cancer, breast cancer, they said that I'd had it two, about two year, you know, they can analyze the growth in it and see how, you know, what type of thing it is. They do all these tests on it and that's what it said, and I said straightaway the voices were telling me that in my head but I couldn't suss it out. 'cos I can remember 'em saying, 'you need help' but I just thought it was 'cos I was a bit doolally at the time, and I never thought anything more about it.... T'finish up I found this lump about here [on the breast] and I went to t'doctors and that's what it turned out to be. Just last year, 12 months ago, and I think to myself I should have found it sooner, you know, if it had been there two year how could I have missed, you know, something as obvious as that.

This narrative fundamentally questions the idea of mental illness and hearing voices as 'irrational' and 'abnormal'. To Rachel there was meaning to her voices, though they were initially overlooked as part of her mental illness. Despite this, Rachel was happy to be compliant with the psychiatrists; there is never a feeling that she blames them for not diagnosing her properly. In fact she is positive about her treatment in psychiatric hospital and the ward staff, and even accepts the psychiatric diagnoses of 'hyper-mania' as the following part of the narrative suggests:

> *A*: 'I'm sure, sure my family don't know what to do with me really. They don't, they don't understand it, but I don't understand it myself. I asked the psychiatrist, he said he, he could understand it.'
> *Q*: 'Right.'
> *A*: 'Which I suppose he's had a lot of experience of people hasn't he?'
> *Q*: 'Umm. Do they give you a label as well, a diagnosis?'

A: 'He said I were "hyper-mania". I suffer from, I suffer from hyper-mania, that's what he called it.'
Q: 'Right. But I guess you sort of see it differently?'
A: 'I don't know, I can't really say because I don't know. I don't want to suffer with it any more anyhow.'
Q: 'Umm. As I say [?] do you still get the voices now then?'
A: 'No, I haven't had any for ages.'
Q: 'Yeah.'
A: 'No, the last August was t'last time that I got them and they wasn't as bad as the first time that I got them. No, I think I'm cured now.'

This part of the conversation may appear rather contradictory after Rachel's narrative linking her illness directly to her undiagnosed breast cancer. But maybe this narrative becomes a 'belt and braces' approach to the illness. Maybe there is not enough 'logicality' that can be attached to such a story and it is as well to have a back-up theory which fits more with conventional wisdom? This suggests that compliance with psychiatry, rather than reacting against the system, can have a positive effect (see Estroff *et al.* 1992). Yet, later on, Rachel reaffirms her original theory and her continued positive attitude:

A: 'Yeah, honest, that's what I think happened to me. And the, the psychiatrists, they don't think that's what it was, you know what I mean, and [the CPN] doesn't think so, you know, have you met [the CPN]? He's a nurse and he comes round to see everybody, he works in [town name].'
Q: 'So he's your CPN?'
A: 'Yeah. And he dun't think it were that, but I do.'
Q: 'Right.'
A: 'And now it's all sorted out, you know, and I've finished with t'treatment and that, I feel alright, I'm cured.'
Q: 'Excellent. So you have an active life again?'
A: 'Yeah, I've started to go dancing, yeah, I'm on the pull when I go out, looking for a new romance.'

Rachel sees the illness as her friend sees it – 'it's only like breaking your leg, it gets better'. She is still taking medication for protection of the ovaries against further cancer scares, but says 'I'd know if there was anything else the matter with [me] 'cos my mind'd tell me now, it, it, I'm sure it'd start and tell me, you know, if there's anything else not right about me'. With this last illumination she moves on to talk about her sons, holidays in Florida and how much she loves food. Before I leave I ask her about the comment of the security guard and what he could have possibly meant. Her ex-husband had just popped up to see her before my arrival, so the security man had obviously made some assumptions as to what I was doing visiting Rachel and looking forward to a colourful outcome.

5.5 Home treatment narrative: Catriona

'I'll do the interview if you can get me out of this place for the day', was roughly how Catriona put it. I had managed to track her down to the local psychiatric hospital where she was currently sectioned (that is, compulsorily detained) – obviously the period with the BHTS had not worked out for her. I had to sign some papers to act as Catriona's 'charge' for the time she was away from the hospital and to promise to bring her back at the end of the day. Sensing my nervousness about the whole situation, Catriona repeatedly makes comments about 'doing a runner' whilst we are in the taxi on the way to the university.

If applying a narrative technique is an attempt to redistribute power in the research situation back to the people being studied, never was this so true as with Catriona. For most of the time during the discussion I feel pretty much out of control of the situation. The interview starts in an office at the university, then we must eat, first in the staff refectory (which Catriona decides against), then in the bar downstairs. After the bar we take a taxi to Catriona's house – which I am very much against but do not want to alienate her – so she can pick up some clothes. The rest of the interview is carried out there. Finally we head back to the hospital a few hours later. By this time my nerves are shot.

Catriona's narrative appears to revolve around some bad relationships with men and the death of her son from a heroin overdose. It is not always clear to me what Catriona is saying because she often seems to follow a stream of thought, and there is often little time for me to be able to clarify points. For instance, what she says of having children is that it,

> Feels like you have them warm and close to you when they're born, and then I got my head beat in, he beat the child as well later on and the child [her son] took drugs and became psychotic, became schizophrenic, so he was lost in the system, checked into [the psychiatric hospital] who had nothing to do with him and just said he was a dump, dirt, a drug addict and if they'd have kept him in there and

> the CPN was supposed to be here, taking him into [the psychiatric hospital] to check, you know, for detox and he never did, he never did it on time, because I kept saying, well the CPN, this CPN told me when I said, he's only twe-, I didn't know how old he was, I thought he was 30, my own son, he was only about 28 and I said to his CPN... is this all right, I said to the CPN, 'well by the time he's 40, he'll still be a young man, let's chip away at this'. The first thing I thought was get him off the bloody injections, you know them, get him off that bloody stuff really slowly and I was saying to him, 'by the time'.... But he knew he were dying and the CPN more or less said, 'well it keeps him off the streets and from robbing'. The CPN knew, but I didn't, I thought there was hope.

It is not clear who the 'he' who beat both Catriona and her child is, but it sounds like her partner. She admits that her son's death 'started it all off'. Since self-referring to hospital she has experienced a lot of what she considers to be negative treatment including medication and compulsory sectioning. Catriona's narrative expresses a lot of anger. For instance, when we talk about the BHTS she says,

> *A*: 'I mean, I really trusted [BHTS staff member] and then he even turned on me, that was Mr paranoia you see, I thought they were coming to get me, well they were coming to get me. They rang up and said, "Oh, we're coming down to see you with your own GP". I didn't ask him to come. I'm with [BHTS consultant], I didn't ask him to come. I'm with [BHTS staff member], I thought, "Oh shit, [BHTS staff member]'s in on it now" – "let's get her bloody drugged, she's got stepping out of order here, she isn't strong enough for all this, she's not gonna be strong enough, we'll help her out by putting the antipsychotic in her" – and that's when my pride and my dignity was hurt and that's when I packed a bag, but first, initially when I went into hospital, I'm going, backtracking now when I initially, I started packing and when the ballistic bag got bigger and bigger. "Ballistic"'s my favorite word you see, when the bag got bigger and bigger and then I start, at about more or less that size of ballistic note writing, I thought "wow wee, what we got here? All psychosis creeping up on you again". I've got one way of summing it up. Psychosis didn't creep up on me, six years ago I stumbled on it. That's a very important thing I've just told you.'
>
> *Q*: 'Yeah, can you explain that a bit more?'
>
> *A*: 'Oh, if I want to.'

Q: Okay.

A: 'If you go on a diet because you've been rejected by your boyfriend who's got somebody new who's slim and beautiful, then women can often go on – what do you call it? – ballistic slimming and ballistic depression as well. "Ballistic" means real big depression, yeah, and real big slimming, 'till after about a fortnight I must have lost half a stone, right, but I started noticing I was getting energy, sorry, getting loads and loads of energy, and I couldn't sleep, you see it started the chemicals going, right, 'cos I wasn't eating properly, and then the big one, the big one where I thought I could paint at a hundred miles an hour and write, and I could for about a few days until the penny dropped and then it turned it to rubbish. But, us people who are called "manic depressions" have a gift that they'd like stamped out, really stamped out, they'd like to be finished with it, they're spending millions and millions and billions on drugs to drug us and they're just scapegoating us, they're just using us. It's a... the picture's bigger than you think.'

At the same time as Catriona is expressing anger about staff betraying her trust, she is also acknowledging the 'psychoses' and 'paranoia' she has 'stumbled' on. The packing of the bags seems to be a way of keeping some control over her situation. Whilst we are doing the interview she is looking through a bag she has with her and, later at the house, she packs some additional things and takes some extra bags with her. As she has already commented, when the staff came for her she began 'packing'. She later describes 'Mr paranoia' as representing 'not trusting you' – when 'Mr Paranoia' appears she is less likely to trust someone. The depression and paranoia is now seen as caused by the boyfriend who left her for another woman. She moves on to tell me that the BHTS would be better if somebody like myself was in charge and there were no psychiatrists involved, 'so that you can say, "well look, please I really feel this person isn't gonna make it without some help, medication help, so could you please prescribe the most gentle, startling gentle...".' Catriona feels that the psychiatric system has not been 'gentle' with her. She expresses a need for some help with her problems, but not the current form of psychiatric treatment:

> People ought to be able to check into the hospital, say, 'look, I'm checking in, for Christ's sake have you got a crying room, a padded room, with a lovely padded bed on it, not things shaken up, all pale

> pink', okay I know what I'm saying. Say this office [at the university] was done out in all beautiful pink soft, so you could just fall asleep. Yeah, and then you could step outside of it like this (opens door)... and you'd have somebody waiting there, and then you could go back in it (closes door) like that, and if the person and then somebody would say, 'are you hungry now?', I'd say, 'god I am', and even though I were babbling (makes babbling noise), babbling, babbling right fast like that, let 'em babble. It's only if they pick some'at sharp up, to hurt somebody, like if I started beating you now right, or, beating themselves or, extreme pain....

When she shows me her bedroom she comments,

> *A*: 'Now here's the ballistic circle bedroom. There's the psychosis. That's what sent me to hospital, just that. Fucking idiots, eh. That's what they bloody thought I was psychotic for.'
>
> *Q*: 'Why? Just 'cos, like, your room was, like, untidy?'
>
> *A*: 'Yeah and my whole house was like this.'

Again, Catriona rejects the labels that psychiatry are using to control her. As she wanders around the house she reiterates her anger and frustration – 'you see how much they hurt me, keeping me in there [psychiatric hospital]?' She describes what she needed from psychiatry as '[staff member from the BHTS] and TLC (tender loving care)'. The significance of the BHTS member of staff is that this person had suffered bereavement and was from a Muslim background. Catriona perceives the Muslim faith as supporting family solidarity in times of crisis. Catriona tends to emphasize her lack of time alone to grieve for her own bereavement(s) and the interruption of psychiatry in her life. Knowing she has to return to the psychiatric hospital later in the day, she becomes intensely angry with psychiatry again:

> They're not just in danger of destroying my mind by hurting me, they're in danger – I don't know if you've got this [tape recorder] running – they're in danger of destroying my whole family and in the end I could lose my house over them, but I'll tell you what, I'll swing. If they do that to me, I will burn myself in front of them, metaphorically speaking. I'm not suicidal, but I'll fucking hurt myself if they do that to me.... So you are the only one that knows now aren't, and [BHTS staff member], the damage they can do. That's... I'm a classic case of damage that can be done and did you know, have

> you read a book called 'Seduction of Madness' [written by Edward M Podvoll]?... In that it will tell you that the patient hasn't got the chemical upset, the damage they can do shoving the chemicals in, have you read about that?

On this grim statement we head back to the hospital. It is easy to assume that Catriona has too much anger and frustration with the psychiatric system to be able to recount a life outside of it in any detail. It is difficult to tell what the illness consists of anymore; if it was originally bereavement of various kinds that lead to the depression, it seems subsumed in the narrative beneath a fury and lack of trust in others.

5.6 Hospital narrative: Tariq

This narrative interview was carried out by the bilingual researcher in Punjabi – Tariq's preferred language. Tariq's narrative reflects a social history similar to many first-generation Pakistanis who settled in Bradford in the 1960s and 1970s. After a number of questions and answers about the interview, the story unravels. Tariq was born in Kashmir, Pakistan. In 1976 – when he was 12 or 13 years old – he came to Britain. He went to school for only two or three years, but learnt to speak English. In 1981 he married a woman who was also from Pakistan. Tariq worked in building maintenance, as he explains,

> Electrical work, like boilers, and with the engineers I used to go round, you know, all the schools in Bradford. If they had a boiler problem or if there was a lift problem anywhere, we'd go and sort it out. Sometimes it was in an office. After that I worked in Morrisons [supermarket] for about four or five years and then after that I was doing these [employment] schemes and things. Community programs, working with the council. Most of the time, been on a [job] training schemes, trying to get job.

He calculates that the last time he was on a training scheme was about two years ago, 'but when you're been on so many schemes as well, you want a job'. Matters turn to the first time he was admitted to hospital:

> *A*: 'You mean, when I was first ill? Well actually I don't really know myself. I was sitting here eating. I was here with my children, my wife, my mother was here, my sisters, my wife's sister was here, and I just got up and started to hit everybody.'

Q: 'You got angry?'
A: 'I was just overtook. Something overtook me.'
Q: 'Do you remember it?'
A: 'I can remember, whatever, you know, like things what I was doing or saying. But, like, something was saying to me "do this" and I was doing it. And I started hitting my, you know, like throwing my kids all over, and started hitting 'em, and my brother came and I started hitting him as well. I was saying that "I've got more power than you lot, everybody, I've got more power than everybody". Then I was mentioning, like at that time, it was in my mind they were like, 666. You know, all the time. And then my neighbor came in and he had a car, it was just the number was 868, and I just didn't like him. He came and I started beating him as well.'
Q: 'What was this number 666, in your head? Where did that come from?'
A: 'Well, just evil. I dunno, why? Just because like, you know, like I, me and my wife, I got five daughters and one son. Just I think...'

Tariq did not recognize the number 666 as meaning anything to him. He could not explain this behaviour, but felt as though his body had been taken over:

> I wouldn't stop. I had no power to stop... Someone was using my body and it's like... I was speaking a person's voice as well, different people's voice. I was speaking, you know, like when I was speaking it was different peoples' voice.

Despite Tariq's feeling that he had no power over his behaviour at this time, he mentions speaking aloud about the arrival of his son, his brother and finally the police, who all appeared after he had announced their arrival. He was fighting with all of them and was finally handcuffed by the police. There are elements of the 'seer' or prophet throughout Tariq's narrative, though he sees this as quite a negative attribute. In seeking to find an explanation for his original outburst against his family and the police he says,

> I can't explain it but it's something, like I can't explain why it happened to me and why did it happen. Like sometimes, still I have dreams, and I have, like, you know, if I have dreams, when I have dreams, if I tell somebody they come true. That's why I don't tell anybody.

Tariq is concerned that making these dreams real for people will have a negative affect on their future. He comments that 'something in my mind is telling me "you mustn't tell them".' If he does not tell people what was in his dreams, then things will work out fine for them. He still cannot explain his behaviour, emphasizing that none of his friends or relatives have had any problems like this and he himself was not depressed or stressed out before this event. After being handcuffed,

> The police took me to a [police] station and then I started saying to them somebody was doing voodoo on me. I said my neighbors across the road are doing it, my next door neighbors are doing it. I mentioned to them that I thought other people had done voodoo on me. And then they had a special doctor and he came and checked me, and I said to him as well that they're doing voodoo on me. And I told him that somebody was making my children and my wife sit down and doing something to them. And that they had dolls and they were sticking pins into them.

Again, there is the feeling of being out of control in this narrative, that others have control of the body. To regain control, there was a need to 'reverse' the situation, as Tariq notes of his subsequent hospitalization,

> I stayed for one night. And that one night was like a nightmare for me. And there were like, unexpected things going on in the hospital, things that I couldn't even have imagined before. I was in the hospital and I got up and I started setting the tables and the knives and forks on the table. This should be here, that should be here, that should be here. I don't know why... I wasn't in control. It was like somebody was making me get up and starting to do things. And I kept thinking that 'if I do this thing then everything will be alright'. It was like, everything had to be... you know normally people go forward? I was thinking I had to reverse everything.

Tariq's feeling was that if anyone 'did anything' to him, he had to reverse it. Yet at the same time as he was carrying out what he himself was seeing as bizarre behaviour, 'I was thinking, "I'm not mad, so why am I doing these things?".' He remains quite powerless throughout this narrative – there are no happy endings for Tariq, as he remains unable to explain his behaviour and he does not perceive himself as being particularly 'better' now. After a period in hospital, he was allowed to go home on the condition that he committed no more acts of violence. Unfortunately, he repeats his earlier behaviour two weeks later. As an explanation he states, 'I lost my memory completely. All I could remember was my wife and my children and my parents. Everything else I completely forgot. All I could remember was my childhood. That was the only thing I could remember'. Gradually his memory came back, though he still has problems with remembering things. Further to this he states,

> The doctor's have given me medicine, so I just take that. But if I don't take that, if I take it I feel drowsy. I feel drowsy, I feel like going to sleep. But if I don't take it, I dunno, I try to not take it but I don't feel comfortable, I just start, I can't sit down, keep moving about all the time.

Tariq also mentions that if he does not take the medicine he starts 'thinking about things more'. He visits psychiatric outpatients every two or three months to see a psychiatrist for a few minutes – he says he feels better when he talks to the psychiatrist but he doesn't know why this is. Unlike Philip's narrative (see Section 5.2), Tariq has no explanation for his behaviour, he is not sure what to do about it, and he also thinks people are looking at him:

> *A*: 'I don't know what to do. Keep thinking, like, people think I'm stupid, you know. Like, if I'm walking, I keep putting my hand in my pocket, other pocket, then I keep taking it out, and things like that.'
> *Q*: 'Do you think people are looking at you?'
> *A*: 'Yeah, that's what I keep thinking. Keep looking, and they're thinking, you know, something wrong with me or summat.'

Tariq states that he does not talk about his problems with anyone apart from the psychiatrists, and this includes his family. However, he soon mentions that his faith and beliefs can be of some use in helping him. First he says, 'now, I don't know if English people will understand, but my mum brought holy charms for me. I've tied holy charms onto my neck and arm – with that I feel better. I've got them on me'. He continues,

> We Muslims, we believe that many things could have happened. Somebody could have done magic on me or put some kind of spell on me. But I don't believe that anybody's done that to me, from the family. But I don't know why at that time, I was saying 'somebody's

> done this on me, somebody's done some magic on me'. I was saying at that time, but I don't really believe that anybody had done any magic on me.

In light of the illness and in seeking explanation, Tariq and his family read the Koran regularly and tend to pray more often:

> I've been reading the Koran every day. The chapter called 'Ya-Sin' every day. The chapter called 'Al-Baqarah', those kind of things. Some people have said 'read these chapters'. Or 'read the chapter called Ya-Sin 40 times, blow on water and then drink the water. Do that for 40 days'. And I've done that as well.

This has made a difference to Tariq in that it has brought him some peace of mind. Yet one cannot help detecting some despair within his narrative. He feels he has changed as a person – that his whole personality has altered since he developed the illness those seven months ago. He comments that he used to laugh but no longer does, he feels nervous when he is with other people now and says very little, so as to not appear 'daft' or show that something is 'wrong with me'. Significantly, he highlights his first night in hospital as the point at which he 'changed'. 'I changed over night,' he says, though still lost as to an explanation as to why he changed. Though he feels the staff did everything they could to help him, he did not feel like a psychiatric patient or that he belonged in hospital.

Tariq sees a '50 per cent improvement' on the time when he was 'really bad' but he still feels there is something wrong with him. He still gets nightmares and can sometimes wake up sweating, even during the winter. Nevertheless, he remains insightful about his illness, commenting,

> I know I'm not daft. But I know, whatever happened to me, I can't, I haven't recovered from the illness. That's what's wrong with me. I keep thinking like, if like, I keep moving, keep making movements, I can't sit down. If I'm sitting like this I keep thinking I should be sitting like this, I shouldn't be sitting like that, I should be sitting like this. And you know, I keep thinking I feel, I don't feel comfortable, you know, like when a lot of people sitting down, like four or five people sitting down, I don't feel comfortable. I keep thinking, you know, when somebody moves, I think 'oh, how should I sit now?', you know what I'm saying?

This narrative has lasted 90 minutes (there are about 20 pages of text), yet it is disappointing to me, as it must be to Tariq, to find that there is no golden nugget or great self-discovery that will 'save' him from his continued bewilderment. Yet as Denzin (1997) has implied, it is the nature of such narratives to be open-ended. I wonder what the psychiatric answer was. True, Tariq is not harming anyone anymore (though he needs continued support from his family), but he is left to recover on his own (if that is possible in this case.). His future aspirations are relatively straightforward: 'first of all I want to recover from my illness. Then . . . gonna do, try to find a job, work . . . obviously. Can't cope with the social money or anything. It's bad, you know'. Though I would not want to pigeonhole Tariq's illness as culturally different simply because he has a Pakistani background, there is always the possibility that the illness makes little sense to us because of our Western model of illness behaviour, rather than a more sociocentric view of illness (these issues will be explored further in Chapter 7).

5.7 Home treatment narrative: Yunas

The narratives reproduced in this chapter so far have skirted around psychiatric treatment and the nature of the institution. Within Yunas's narrative, the psychiatric institution takes centre stage. Due to the effects of hospital treatment, very little is learnt about Yunas's history before this period. Only with the intervention of home treatment and support from his family is he able to consider a future without psychiatry. Yunas spends a lot of time talking about the home treatment team's intervention with him and his family, often noting that he feels they did everything they could for him including changing his GP, significantly lowering the amount of medication he was taking and spending extended periods of time with him at his home. But the positive aspects of home treatment are in stark contrast to the hospital care he received. Yunas himself feels that the illness he was suffering from initially,

> Was more of a depression, the state that I was in, it wasn't more of a manic depression or anything of that nature. It was just acute depression. But they stopped classing it as a psychosis. And obviously once you fall into the hands of the hospital they have to treat that. You understand what I mean. And that is what kind of situation I fell into. And they [home treatment] pulled me out of it.

He describes the difference between home treatment and hospital care as,

> The complete opposite of each other. Home treatment service listen to what you've got to say. They work off what you've got to say. It's, whoever's not listening they'll stick up for you and tell 'em, they speak on your behalf. And the hospital's completely the opposite. They get the information off the doctor and just pump drugs into you.

Yunas felt that he was used as a 'guinea pig' by the hospital, being forcibly given medication against his will. He had asked the doctors to lower his medication but to no avail. He explains this within the context of his first two occasions of hospitalization:

> The first two times I was, two months and one month and then another month, it changed my whole life completely, gave me nightmares and rest of it, never used to have no nightmares. And the side effects [of the drugs] are vicious, vicious, tremors, you've no, I, I'd no control over my brain. I didn't, it wasn't me I didn't feel as if it was me controlling my brain, the drugs were controlling my brain. It was, it was just, and on one occasion they did give me a high dose and I had an epileptic fit, never been epileptic in me life... And the drugs. Later on I picked a dictionary, three years later, a medical dictionary, one of me cousins brought me it. Started reading through, and reading all the side effects, and they, the list's like that in a small... book, the list's full pages full of warnings and side effects. They didn't take, no one would take no notice of anything of that nature before they, you know, put them drugs inside us.

But this was not the only form of institutional violence that Yunas experienced during his initial periods of hospitalization. Yunas explains that some of the staff were prone to physical violence and threatening behaviour. Many complaints were made by users, but 'they never seemed to get through'. He illustrates this by commenting on his first time in hospital:

> *A*: 'When I first went in there [psychiatric hospital] I was attacked by one of the staff. Had me arm, I went, I went to hospital for x-rays as well 'cos he pulled me.... He wanted me to stay in me room and I wanted to speak to somebody from me family. I wanted to use

the phone and he wouldn't let me, wanted me to stay in me room and he jumped on me, pulled me arm up me back and kept me head down like that, and put, putting his knee on me back. And on one occasion someone, someone kicked an exit door open or pushed an exit door open. Then I went outside and sat on a bench, why I don't know ... very strong tranquillizer at the time, injection. I wandered out the door and the man who'd done that gets away with it all, they tie me down, pinned me down. And bruises, foot marks, I had foot prints, me family come to see me I had foot prints on me shoulders, these scars are still visible now, to this day. Foot print marks on me back. I was bruised here and there.'

Q: 'Because you wandered out these open doors?'

A: 'Just wandered out, and I, it wasn't me it was the drugs. What I'm trying to say, there is no, the hospital do not look after you properly, whereas home treatment service do. They're completely the opposite. They [hospital staff] just give you your drugs, that's all that's their concern – to keep you inside that ward, that is it.'

It is unsurprising given these experiences of institutionalization that Yunas's narrative centres around the effects of the violence and forced medication. He had no control over his situation. Yunas's family complained about the state they would find him in when they visited, but this does not seem to have had a lot of effect in Yunas's opinion. His hopes were kept alive by praying and knowing that his family were also praying for him, hoping he would get out of hospital one day and get back to his 'normal self'. If there is a classic narrative of the hospital creating illness within people then this is it: though it is hard to determine what was wrong with Yunas before hospital, once he was in hospital, the 'illness' really started to show itself. As he notes, 'when you're heavily tranquillized ... I started having paranoid illusions and the rest of it. So it was just, just a whole nightmare for me'. We do get a little insight into the person Yunas used to be before hospitalization when he says of his younger days that he was,

A: 'Young, confident, a very young confident young man I was. Wasn't, no fears you know, no nothing. In there [psychiatric hospital], when they started putting them drugs they seem to completely take over you, they paralyzed me. I used to feel as if me brain was paralyzed as well. And then all the paranoid illusions and all that comes into it. You just end up confusing someone who's talking normally to you, you end up confusing them, 'cos you're just imagining things, and I didn't know I were imagining it. I actually thought they were real and they weren't.'

Q: 'Right, so you end up not knowing what's real and what's not?'

A: 'Mmm, until the drugs stopped. Then I woke up, you know, you understand what I mean.'

The word 'paralyzed' is also a useful metaphor for what has happened to Yunas's life since first coming into contact with psychiatry. Most of all, he blames his first GP for diagnosing him as 'psychotic'. Yunas feels this was wrong: 'there was never no psychotic behavior come from me. I never harmed no one. Never tried to harm myself.' Since this first diagnosis, Yunas has been given a variety of labels from different doctors (including 'schizophrenia', 'psychotic', 'manic depression', 'schizophrenia with manic depression', and finally 'a bit of depression') and they have all served to undermine his self-identity and his self-confidence. He now has a feeling of having to 'watch my own back all the time' and be ready for any possible 'relapse'. Only through breaking free of the drugs and hospital is Yunas once again able to take some control over his own life, though the following conversation illustrates the difficulties in reintegrating with others:

Q: 'And since you've come out of hospital, do you think you've been able to get back to where you were, you know, right at the beginning?'

A: 'No way, no way. Lost me, I haven't lost me friends but it's hard for 'em, for me to go off and socialize. I can't, I've lost me socializing skills, confidence.'

Q: 'What do you mean you've lost them?'

A: 'Well I can't, I can't socialize, I used to be able to blend in with anybody, talk to anyone, get on with 'em and the rest of it. I just don't, happen no more, I'm more of a lonely person now.'

Q: 'Right, you find it more difficult to sort of, create friendships?'

A: 'Yeah.'

Q: 'Why do you think that is?'

A: 'That, that experience I've had in hospital. Just knocked everything out of me.'

Q: 'It's like your confidence has been damaged?'

A: 'Yeah. Felt as if I was gonna end up dead. After the epileptic seizure bit, that were it. I, I, just, I thought I were, I thought I was gonna pass away, the way I felt. And from there it's just, you know, it took it's time.'

As was outlined earlier in this narrative, Yunas was given tranquillizers that gave him epileptic fits. He was also told by the staff that the effect of the drug would wear off after three days. What they did not tell him – what he later found out from his dictionary of medicine – is that the drug actually remains in the system for around 18 months. He lost count of the number of injections he was given, but obviously feels worried that he will experience more fits or some other kind of a relapse due to this medication. This has particularly damaged his self-confidence, and scares him when he thinks about the future and possibly going back to work. He states later that he needs his

> Self-confidence back, that's the main thing. The main, when I used to go for job interviews – I mean, I've got a job record, always in work – and it was me confidence that used to get me through interviews, and get me in work and keep me going in work, get me going. You know, you understand what I mean?

Now that he has lost this self-confidence and belief in himself it is difficult to get it back, although he received some encouragement from the home treatment team, his CPN and his family. He also mentions that he is attempting to get back to playing football and socializing more with his friends. 'I enjoyed football', he says, 'it's a good exercise and I play, I play well. I play very well, I get a lot of satisfaction out of scoring goals. That's what I was doing before I went in to hospital.'

When we talk of 'illness' and 'periods of crisis' it is assumed that we are talking about the individual's personal problems, yet Yunas's narrative reminds us that this may not be the case at all. Whatever Yunas's problems were before seeing his local GP, they were subsequently subsumed under the much larger crisis caused by hospitalization. Finally, Yunas highlights what he believes should change in hospital psychiatry:

> Discipline the staff. Have regular check-ups with patients, talk to patients in private rooms. Listen to what they've got to say, act on that, on, on their information. Visit staff, have words with them. Talk to the GPs, family psychiatrist, to monitor the drugs, side-effects and so on.

5.8 Hospital narrative: Carmen

Early morning, the odd bit of drizzle about, but generally not too bad. I leave on foot for Carmen's house which is about a kilometre away.

Not a bad spot, you can see quite a lot of green about and the town of Shipley in the distance. I arrive not too wet. Carmen's husband answers the door of the council house and I am soon fixed up with a cup of tea. I feel a bit guilty because they are still in the middle of their breakfast (they have no telephone, so I wrote ahead hoping they would be there for my visit). Both Carmen and her husband stick around whilst I am there. Any thoughts that this might impede Carmen is quickly washed aside by her assertiveness. The exchanges that take place between her and her husband are also very interesting, as they often give different views of the medical and personal encounters they've experienced.

In contrast to Tariq, Carmen's narrative tells us much about the medical profession's changing knowledge base and its dealings with individuals perceived as being 'sick' or in need of medical intervention. For instance, the first thing she tells me is,

> I were born epileptic fits, right, and for years the doctors had been trying to make me take medication and stuff like that and I've been always fighting against it. Because to be put on, well they called amphetamines back then, they were basically speed, and I was only I think about three or four, you know, as young as that and to be having that sort of treatment....

The doctors have tried to put Carmen on other drugs for her epilepsy but she has remained unsure of the benefits of medication, and of the doctors who prescribe them. She contemplates the dangers of professionals with such power when she says, 'of course you're not getting into what the doctors are doing, you just put your kids and folks into their hands, but it's not always the best policy'. It is not just the side effects of the medication that have had a negative effect on her opinion of doctors (she experienced multiple epileptic fits after taking one particular form of medication), but also the 'sickness' label that she appears unwilling to accept. As she says of gaining employment, 'there's no point in me going for interview and telling the people [about the epilepsy] because you know what the answer's going to be – they're not going to give you a job'. The epilepsy has cost her a number of jobs in the past because of periods off work or the fits coming on during work and putting herself in danger. For her own safety, Carmen's husband would like her to stay at home, though she reasons that she is in no less danger in the house – where she may be cooking or running a bath when the next fit happens (as has been the case in the past).

I am beginning to wonder how this narrative links to her mental health experiences. Carmen comments on the different names the medical profession have given her epilepsy over time:

> I feel as though what's happened is the name has gone from 'epileptic fit', 'cos everybody who had fits, at one stage of some form, whether it were mild or strong, they were all pushed into that category, it were an 'epileptic fit'. And so as, as I've got older and, depending on who the different fancy names out there, you know, you see, well now they've come up with this fancy title – 'Vasavable [?] Syndrome'.

Carmen explains that she had had a lot of miscarriages (she felt some had been caused by the medication) and, together with the epilepsy, she ended up at psychiatric hospital for a short while. She comments,

> They say that it's, it was a breakdown but I don't know what they're meaning by 'breakdown', I don't know how, what, how they've diagnosed as that. Because when I've seen people... working with people that have had children or they haven't had any, now it's when they become obsessed, they're either going to go one way or the other. Like I've never, I've never, no matter how many miscarriages I've had – and if the truth be known I've had quite a few – I mean I think it must be, with the twins, it must be 12 or ten, I'll have a quick count up... yeah, about ten. But I've never become to the point of obsessive, I just sort of have a – not that I don't care – I have a carefree attitude. There's a difference in that, but not to the point where I say, 'come on [husband's name] we must work all these hours, and we must go and see if we could get these treatments to have children, or we must go and steal somebody's children', you know. So, no I've never been to that extreme or, you know, but it depends, it's the extremes people go to for what they want. You know, as I say I'm just happy, I just think, 'well it's just life and I'm just happy going through it', you know.

Carmen had a series of epileptic fits one particular Thursday, which led to the miscarriage of twins she was carrying. She had been doing a business course at college; her husband blames the pressure of the course for the fits coming on. Carmen does not blame her studies, though she does admit to missing driving in her car. Due to the danger of driving, she was walking instead and realizes now that she must have been finding it wearing. She explains the process of recovering from an epileptic fit:

> I know when you have a seizure, like, that you invest a whole day to recuperate, you know, you do need a whole day to recuperate because it's like this, this, it's like somebody getting into your body and taking over. Well I can't really say a person, but some sort of energy that gets in and you've gone into this fit. So the brain has shot off and it's like the heart is not sending enough oxygen, blood to the brain, so you've gone into this state.

Her husband found her behaviour very unusual at this time and – although he admits she does 'race away' with things sometimes – he had not seen his wife so 'up and down' and acting so strange as he did in the days following the miscarriage. He was at a loss as to what to do, and decided she needed some time at the psychiatric hospital (though he now regrets this):

> Well, I mean, I thought that he [husband] said we were going to the hospital but, so I don't, and I know sometime when you come back from a seizure like what had happened and your body is still functioning but it's like all the little circuits haven't connected back up after a fit like that, you know, you've slapped your head or whatever. And you are, you are in a way disorientated, that is what I would say what happens... It was atrocious, 'cos they knew that I didn't want to take any of the medication, and they had to wait until he [husband] turned up, and they had to wait until he turned up for me to take the medication. I mean like the first days or so they would use injection.

As a result of the drugs she felt sedated, weak and drowsy. Carmen was diagnosed by the psychiatrist as suffering from 'hypomania'. She had never heard of the diagnosis before, although she perceives herself as being 'hyperactive'. It seems in suffering the after-effects of this severe attack she was manifesting symptoms seen as confirmation of a mental illness. For instance, she explains of her state at the time,

> I was still, with having those two attacks at the, cos when you get these multiple fits like that it's like you've been electrocuted in a way, you've been shot at. You know, you've gone into this coma state and you know that something's coming around after the coma, you know, it's a while you're trying to get back to thinking where

> you are, you want to recognize, to be, so they say and you do need a few days to recuperate, but to be, but everything were just sort of rushed up (laughing), it was so my mind couldn't settle down. So everyone, you know, everyone sort of, even when I was speaking, if I was speaking, I was exciting but that's how, that's just me, it looked, so according to my husband, other people, they said that I were like a record player playing at two different speeds, right, because it's like the mind is so far ahead and the mouth always try to keep up with the mind, but it doesn't always (laughing), but that's not wrong either.

After two weeks, Carmen had recovered from the shock of the miscarriage, the fits and the medication. She stayed in hospital for another three weeks, but adds that for most of this period she was back at home with her husband and sometimes not returning to the psychiatric hospital until the following day. She continues to be optimistic about her life and her epilepsy, and seems unconcerned about the labels she was given by the medical profession. She sees parts of her experience in the psychiatric hospital as a learning process, where she was also concerned to help other users. She says at one point,

> You look at yourself and you look at other people around who are labeled as disfigured, right. 'cos I gotta say that I'm disfigured in a sense that my symptoms, they're invisible but they become visible if you know what I'm saying.

I wasn't quite sure what she was saying but I think that it might be that her 'illness' (that is, the epilepsy) is made visible by the medical intervention there has been, which is then carried around within her and has become part of her psyche. Obviously, Carmen has already had to adapt at home and work to avoid the 'showing' of her illness. She is obviously aware of her many miscarriages – which have at least in part been due to the epilepsy – and she is able to accept the illness as a part of her being, rather than seeing it as something that she should be afraid of or reject. As she says of the incidents leading up to hospitalization,

> The only thing, the problem with myself was I miscarried, that's a big thing, and I just needed time to rest, you know. And 'cos it took a lot out of my body and I just needed time to rest. But I wasn't, I wasn't allowed that and, as well, I didn't really allow myself the TV because I couldn't, with all this, with having these multiple attacks at the time, it's as if people just get, well they had to be there, they

> had no choice, I had to be round. Even if they didn't, even if they didn't help me, you know, it probably make them feel safer, they felt though they were doing right. Whereas probably I'd have been better off being left on my own (laughing), you know, and get on with it, you know. And everything just exploding, and I could see, I could see why it's not, that I'm coloring it because I think [the psychiatrist] got the impression that I were in denial. And I says 'no, I've had this condition and these are the responses that do happen'.

Carmen is still planning on finishing her college course and then following it up by undertaking a degree course in Plymouth. Her husband, meanwhile, was released from his job and put on 'the sick' to be able to care for his wife (who he is still worried about). Her husband continues to appear more concerned about Carmen's illness than she does herself. Carmen analyzes her own behaviour at the time of being hospitalized and what she was trying to communicate to people. She admits,

> It was strange, and, 'cos I know when I'd mentioned things to [the psychiatrist] about people being into this sort of voodoo and witchcraft, and they think that I were wanting to be this person or something. And, like, that word 'reincarnation', now as far as I'm concerned that word 'reincarnation' is how people, the definition. Because to me 'reincarnation' in my head it means similar, it doesn't mean, if you're not putting it into a religious thing. Like I know that if you look at it from a religious point of view that word 'reincarnation' can sound like a rebirth or a recycle, right. But if you take it from that aspect, there are people who look similar or they have similar temperaments. Am I making sense? But it's how they, it's how they, and how they, 'cos it were, like, with doing this course they do bring about more newer words because you're always learning. Every day you're learning something. And it's how people define these words and where they're labeling it to. 'cos I think that is what when he [husband] say I were 'babbling', I wasn't fully aware of what I were talking about, but just that they couldn't keep up with my mind. And it were wrong to expect them to at the time, but because the situation had got well out of control (laughing), but I find it funny, so now they have to fit all the bits back together.

The idea of 'fitting all the bits back together' would seem to reflect the Western model of psychiatry that attempts to explain perceived patterns of behaviour. Carmen is unsure herself, hence asking me if she is making any sense. Yet her narrative as a whole does make sense. The major questions are of medicine, not of her behaviour. It does not appear that psychiatry did much for Carmen; she did not expect it to. Nevertheless, she is concerned to try and understand what she is doing when she is ill with the epilepsy and how her body changes, and to make sense of these changes within herself. It would seem a mistake that Carmen ended up hospitalized in the first place but, luckily, the experience has not had a negative effect on her general social narrative.

5.9 Home treatment narrative: Raiza

Raiza was born in Bangladesh and then raised in Bradford (the interview was, again, carried out by our bilingual researcher). When she was 15 years old she had what she describes as a 'nervous breakdown':

> I actually had long, quite long hair and I cut it . . . I didn't know what I was doing with myself and my mum was really mad, and when she saw me she got quite a shock. I felt that one part of my head was getting really heavy and my hair was weighing it down so I wanted to cut it, thinking that if I lost the weight of my hair then my head would be back to normal. But, I don't know, it didn't really help. At that time I was feeling that the left part of my body wasn't as good as the right part of my body is, you know . . . like good and bad. Things like that. It was all mixed up in my mind. I didn't know what I were doing.

She relates her breakdown very much to her thoughts and feelings about school and her family at the time:

> At school I was being, not bullied as such, but I was a quiet person, and I thought that I was being walked over and I didn't know how to say anything to them. I mean, I'm not the sort of person that will say anything to them, more like a doormat and they walked all over me. And there was another person, a boy actually, he used to make remarks about him and me . . . you know, like boys do at that age, having a baby together and things like that. And I couldn't handle it. And there were a few occasions when I actually cried at school and took my dad to see some . . . and he got a telling off and had to apologize kind of thing, but that was one or two of the things that . . . The other thing was, my whole life I didn't feel that much part of the family and I felt that . . . I mean my mum and dad hadn't

> done anything to make me feel this way but I felt that just being at a school and all these, you know, like my peers, kind of thing, and I felt that I was being pressured into being more of a proper Muslim and I was rebelling against that idea. That was one of the reasons, and I hated myself afterwards for it but at the time I couldn't help the way I felt.

The feelings of being a 'doormat' at school, not being a 'proper Muslim' or a full part of the family are also contextualized within Raiza's feelings about herself. She quite openly admits that she 'wanted a bit more freedom. I mean, a lot of girls go through that stage in their lives anyway and it's hard to overcome that, but eventually you do'. Due to her breakdown, Raiza spend a period of time at a child and adolescent unit, and consequently left school without any qualifications. She cites the periods of significance for her since then as being her trip to Bangladesh with her sister – during which her sister got married – her varied training and employment experiences and, relatively recently, getting married and having a baby. She is now 25 years old.

Raiza has had periods of illness to varying degrees over the last ten years and it is interesting the way her problems have seemed to change over time, especially from a feeling of well-being in having periods away from home and the family to the point more recently where she has sometimes found it very difficult even to leave the house. This is illustrated by her positive comments about her time at the child and adolescent unit, which she describes as a 'home away from home'. Here she had drama and art therapy, group therapy with the involvement of nurses and psychiatrists as well as activities in smaller groups such as occasionally making tea for everyone at the unit. Raiza felt she had gained responsibility and confidence from her period at the unit, and was treated almost like a member of staff at times, helping to organize activities for others. She comments on her period at the unit and the transition back to home life,

> [At the unit] there were horses and there were stables just next door to the house, and we could see some horses in the field, and sometimes we would go and feed them bread and stuff. It was nice. I mean, for me it was like something out of a story, you know.... It was nice while it lasted. It was hard when I came back home because... not that I wasn't given much freedom, but it was different you know, I had to settle back into being home again... but things... I was a different person for a while, because I had a lot more confidence in me than

> I thought. And I wasn't so aware because I was very paranoid, and my instincts, people were always talking and things like that. Like you do, when you, you become too anxious about things and you get a bit paranoid. It helped me to overcome my.... They did say that I'd become a stronger person.

Raiza comments that when she went to Bangladesh she stopped taking the prescribed medication for her problems. On her return she saw a doctor, 'because I wasn't so well within myself'. She had been working in temporary employment but gave it up as she again 'was feeling down within myself' and became afraid to leave her house. She explains,

> I didn't step a foot outside the house and I was very paranoid, thinking that people had heard that I wasn't going out of the house and were talking about me, whispering behind my back, saying 'This is what you like get'... and, like, voices in my head kind of thing, almost like whispering. I thought that they were talking about me and that didn't help matters.

The doctor prescribed her some new medication, which – apart from the side effects of drowsiness and weight gain – Raiza found had a considerable positive effect on her health:

> [The medication] helped keep my emotions in balance. I'm not feeling too high, I'm not too low. It sort of, like, dull the voices that I have or the paranoia. It sort of dulls it a little so I'm more... I've got more of a feeling of well-being within myself.

Raiza continues to get support and comfort from her family, yet feels that they do not really understand what she has been going through. She describes her illness as a mixture of 'feeling really low', 'not feeling myself', being 'depressed' and being 'paranoid'. She has got comfort from reading the Koran and from talking to nurses (including those at the BHTS) about her illness. But her prime incentives to get better and stay well surround her immediate family. Firstly, she says of her child,

> I think that, emotionally, having a baby helped me. Now and again I do get quite depressed and having the baby has helped me focus my attention on him and not myself. So I'm not brooding as much as I used to... so having [child's name] is quite good for me I suppose, therapeutic.

Secondly, her husband, who is still in Bangladesh and has yet to see her baby. Her current job is still temporary and, until it is made permanent, they cannot apply for an entry visa for her husband. She obviously feels certain pressures to 'be well' for the sake of her immediate family:

> I mean, sometimes I just like to stay at home and look after the baby, but then I think if I don't go out and get a job my husband will never be over. I feel a bit pressured that way but, in the long run, I don't mind because it makes... certain that I, things get sorted out, the sooner he'll be over and we'll be a proper family.

'The family' has been a key theme throughout Raiza's narrative, as has her perceived struggle for some freedom and to be accepted as a good person. I wonder if these separate parts of her life are not intrinsically related. It would seem the family is now – or maybe it always was? – perceived as stability and order within her life, yet Raiza continues to question herself and her commitment to the values she longs for. For example, she admits at one point, 'sometimes I don't really like myself that much... but I mean overall I think I am quite an all right person. I think people might like to have me as a friend, but then again I don't know'. Then, later, she says of the future,

> The only thing I would like in my future is to be a bit more... religious minded... I hate myself that I never read them all, you know, be more better that way, but at the moment... you know, I should always make time but I don't. I keep myself... that's one thing I'd like to correct.

Despite maintaining a series of jobs, getting married and having a baby as well as coping with the illness, Raiza still finds that the problem lies within herself. When she has been ill, things have not made sense, she has needed the help of others to pull her through. Although she has stated that she has felt stronger and more confident as a result of her life and illness experiences, she maintains at the end of her narrative that 'I don't think I ever have coped really well'.

5.10 Hospital and home treatment user narratives

Given the complexity, diversity and sheer fluidity witnessed within the eight narratives presented, it is naturally a difficult task to detect themes that run through both groups of users to be able to compare narratives.

At the level of professional competence, psychiatry as a whole appears problematic within the user narratives outlined so far. Philip feels he got little help from the system other than the medication; Tariq feels only '50 per cent better' after treatment; Carmen and Rachael are more inclined to see themselves as having suffered physical illnesses; Catriona is very angry at the system as a whole; Yunas was physically abused by staff and medication was administered by force; only Raiza and Michael (both clients of the BHTS) appear to have received anything significant from psychiatry. At the very least, the BHTS is seen by users in a less negative light than hospitalization. This certainly backs up a lot of other studies that compare the two models of care (for example, Fenton *et al.* 1979, 1984; Hoult *et al.* 1983; Muijen *et al.* 1992; Orme and Cohen 2001; Smyth and Hoult 2000; Test and Stein 1980).

The majority of the narratives reproduced in this chapter illustrate the different ways in which psychiatry and similar authorities can exercise power and control over ordinary people, whether through coercive means or through more liberal forms of care such as home treatment. These can include the taking of medication, interventions with users and families, attendance at clinics and outpatients, referral for counselling, CPN input, sectioning and voluntary hospitalization. The dominance of medical psychiatry is such that through reading the user texts we are soon aware of what a likely psychiatric diagnosis and treatment for a user is going to consist of. This is despite the fact that the texts highlight clear extremities and diversities of need. Once in contact with the psychiatric system the narratives are muted in favour of the medical aetiology that talks of 'illness', 'diagnosis', 'treatment', and 'cure'.

Home treatment's place within the psychiatric services is interesting. Being self-defined as an 'alternative' to hospitalization for those suffering acute and severe mental health problems has its advantages. For a number of the users, *any* alternative to hospitalization would be gratefully received. The home treatment user narratives suggest that such alternatives can work for the user and help them in a positive way, for example, reduction in medication levels, allowing people to talk through their problems, as well as dealing with other social and economic problems the user might have (this is perhaps inevitable when working with a user in their own home). There seems to be acceptance that the user's problems cannot be simply seen as 'pathological'. Whereas the hospital narratives show the psychotic labels of 'schizophrenia' and 'manic depression' remain common, the home treatment user narratives refer more to the general diagnosis of 'depression'. This may suggest that the home treatment service is dealing with less 'severe' users, but it could equally mean there is less of an emphasis on psychiatric labels. We can also see from the hospital narratives that two women – Rachel and Carmen – were both given similar psychotic labels, whilst they have personally rejected these in favour of the physical illnesses of cancer and epilepsy, respectively.

Whereas home treatment has taken a liberal approach to the treatment of users, hospital has not wanted to or has not been able to. These narratives talk of hospitalization in terms of authority and control, of biomedical treatment and institutional violence. However, as was mentioned earlier, Estroff *et al.* (1992) have noted that possible acceptance of diagnoses and illness behaviour can have a more positive outcome than those who reject such labelling. It is interesting that those who experienced hospital as being very negative (that is, Philip, Tariq, Catriona, and Yunas) are still having difficulties in progressing with their lives. The other users appear more passive to psychiatric treatment – in whatever form it has been received – and these people seem to have been able to maintain a positive outlook. Consequently, these narratives often look beyond psychiatry and speak of other parts of their lives.

Generally speaking, the narratives open up a labyrinth of ways of experiencing 'illness' and 'health'. As has been suggested throughout this chapter, the two concepts are often inseparable. Though there is usually no specific route 'in' and 'out' of the illness for people – and this may appear to be a rather Western-centric view of 'illness' in itself – we can detect two different forms of perceiving one's illness experience. Firstly, there is the view that there has been temporary discordance with the world (as experienced by Rachael, Carmen and Michael for example) that has now been overcome (or, one could say, a process of 'being cured' has taken place). This would conform to Parsons' (1937) idea of the 'sick role' in which a form of 'social contract' is carried out between doctor and patient, in which both parties accept the other's role in allowing a person to be sick and have time off work, medication and so on. The contract is only broken when a person is not seen to recover and is, thus, violating their economic role in (and for) society. This brings us to the other group of users who are more likely to see themselves as permanently ill, such as Yunas who worries about the possibility of relapse or Tariq who has only half recovered and continues to reflect on what has happened to him. There is no obvious return to the labour market or to being an active citizen for these users; some are noted on the national census as being 'permanently sick'. Their social role – thus their social identity – is diminished. Perhaps for this group a more accurate theory would be Merton's (1957) theory of social action that builds on Parsons' work. Maybe this group understands that they have neither the positive means nor the positive ends to achieve societal goals – such as being economically active – and have instead chosen alternative ways to lead a fulfilling life. The narratives illustrate that these lives are currently in transition and that society's perception of them as 'sick' continues within their own psyche. These issues will be looked at further in Chapter 8.

5.11 Conclusion

This chapter has reproduced eight user narratives as completely as possible, illustrating the individual complexities of illness and recovery behaviour as well as the significant place of psychiatry within all of the texts. It has also been demonstrated as to how one might reproduce 'messy texts' in social science writings. Some reflexivity has been performed by placing the researcher within the research process and in the reproduction of the texts. The narratives show a multiplicity of experience and life accounts. Chapters 6 and 7 will offer complementary analysis of all 49 user texts collected. There are a number of themes that emerge from further analysis: Chapter 6 focuses on the descent into illness and psychiatric treatment, whilst Chapter 7 will investigate routes to recovery and user self-coping techniques.

6
Descent into Illness and Psychiatric Intervention

> I think they're missing the point totally, absolutely. They try to tell me I have a fixation with chocolate because I eat a lot of chocolate, but I know a lot of people that eat a lot of chocolate.
>
> (Gillian)

6.1 Summary

In Chapter 5, eight user narratives were reproduced whilst avoiding the imposition of the author's own subjective meaning onto these stories. Each narrative remained a singular and discursive whole. In this chapter – as well as Chapter 7 – issues that surround illness experience and meaning will be investigated through content analysis of all 49 user texts. The narratives have been 'cut and pasted' together by themes and areas, selections from each text have been made and put side-by-side with other user texts. Some generalizations are made here. Thus, the author's interpretations and influences on the process of analysis are more obvious and to the fore in these chapters. It should be noted, however, that the reporting still attempts to give primacy to the user narratives rather the commentary. Together with the user narratives presented in Chapter 5, these two chapters present a comprehensive picture of experience, treatment and meanings of illness and health for the user.

6.2 Precipitating factors

To understand more about 'illness beginnings' and 'illness trajectories' it is necessary to explore the initial contact between the user and

Table 6.1 Coded responses from user narratives highlighting precipitating factors to original crisis*

	Hospital	Home treatment	Total
Drink or drugs	6	1	7
Family/relationship problems	2	5	7
Family bereavement	3	2	5
Education or work problems	3	2	5
Financial problems	2	0	2
Other factors	8	1	9
Do not know	4	1	5
Not recorded	1	8	9
Total	29	20	49

* Each user has been assigned to one category only.

the psychiatric service. Many users commented on the initial event or process which led to such contact. These parts of the narrative have been coded and itemized for both psychiatric hospital and home treatment users in Table 6.1. The majority of users made a correlation between the start of their illness careers and upsetting or traumatic experiences within their lives. Thus, we can see from Table 6.1 that social and economic issues are seen as precipitating factors in many of the narratives. Family, relationships, work and studies are all significant factors, as are bereavement, drink and drugs. 'Other factors' included physical illness, post-natal depression and attempted suicide. Just one user narrative suggested that the start of their illness might have been caused by a pre-existing neurobiological state.

Some differences between the psychiatric hospital and the BHTS user groups can be highlighted from this analysis, with more family and relationship problems – usually divorce or separation – within the home treatment group appearing to trigger the start of the illness. The hospital group, meanwhile, have more people who felt drink or drugs had triggered their illness. This finding is probably due to the hospital running a detoxification programme; the BHTS were less likely to take alcohol and drug users. Some user narratives suggested a combination of factors led to the illness:

> I had a complete breakdown, me husband walked out on me and it triggered off a compete breakdown. I were taken up by the police, I just trashed the flat. I don't remember doing it but they'd put

> me on.... Prozac, but I were on Synatiadin [?] and another medicine.... [It] made me really aggressive but I didn't realize what were going on. (Gillian)

> It was the pressure of work. I spent all my time thinking about work and I'd no close friends. It was before I was married so I'd nobody really that I could share the things that were worrying me about and just everything seemed to build up and push me over the top eventually. (Tony)

> My dad died... and then we had a great big family fallout and, you know, I just wasn't coping. Plus the dog was going in for a serious operation and my daughter's waiting to go in for a serious operation, so it was just a build-up of everything. (Fiona)

Though these user narratives would seem to support the need for a social model of psychiatric intervention, detractors would rightly point to the many people who suffer qualitatively similar points of distress yet do not call on psychiatric services and do not suffer forms of 'mental illness'. There is still the argument that mental illness is biologically based and set off by points of stress such as those found in Table 6.1. As Anita comments, 'the illness is already there but it's aggravated by... my negative thoughts all the time'. To understand further the illness narrative and the power of psychiatry to reshape the self we need to explore users' experiences of hospital and home treatment psychiatry.

6.3 Referrals

How users are referred to a psychiatrist and, consequently, onto a psychiatric service is straightforward in theory, yet in the narratives appear to be down to chance. People seem to end up in hospital or on home treatment as much through accident as design. Leeroy complained, 'I'd say two or three people out of ten who visit the GP are depressed and... have underlying mental illnesses but get dealt with by their GP. I was unfortunate for it to go on too far and see a consultant which screwed up my life entirely, basically'. Far from there being a system of diagnoses and treatment based on an efficient, equal and fair health bureaucracy and scientific model of care, selection depends very much on agency, custom and practice, medical stereotyping, varied models of psychopathology and the power of those referring. This is demonstrated throughout this section.

A crucial – if maybe obvious – point to make here is that, at the point of crisis, many users feel in need of assistance and sometimes specify that they require psychiatric care. As an example, Brian comments, 'I knew I was ill and I knew I...needed treatment or therapy or you know some form of counseling.' Many of the narratives express similar feelings. After the initial trauma, users begin to feel 'out of control', 'freaked', 'completely gone' or suffering 'a complete nervous breakdown' (for similar examples, see Lapsley *et al.* 2002: 25). Users are brought to the attention of the psychiatric services in a number of ways: sometimes self-referral via a GP, sometimes by family members, and – especially in the case of ethnic minorities – through police intervention. There are also those who entered hospital through a variety of other means. A cluster of female users, for instance, entered psychiatric hospital after a period of time at the local general hospital. Such referrals to psychiatric hospital could come about due to attempted suicide, post-natal depression or following examinations for physical complaints which doctors failed to find a physical basis for. Some referrals bordered on the plain mysterious, as Julie's narrative suggested:

A: 'They put something on me finger...then they put sommat on me ear. Then they just told me to go up to [the psychiatric hospital].'
Q: 'Right, right, and they didn't tell you why. They didn't tell you why they were taking you to...'
A: '...No, no the ambulance just took me up there.'

6.4 Psychiatric hospital

As has been explained earlier, although 20 users had experienced the BHTS as an alternative to psychiatric hospital in their last period of crisis, nearly all of the users (47 out of the 49 users) in the research had previously experienced a period of hospitalization. This section explores institutional practice and treatment of *all* users who had experience of psychiatric hospitalization.

In many cases the user narratives were orientated towards experiences of psychiatric hospital and treatment. An assessment of the negative and positive aspects of the hospital from the texts are summarized in Table 6.2 and developed in the following subsections.

6.4.1 Environment

Jane sums up her hospital experiences like this: 'when it was good it was very, very good and when it was bad it was horrid...I think it's very

Table 6.2 Positive and negative aspects of psychiatric hospital summarized from the user narratives*

	Environment	**Staff**	**Treatment**
Positive	Make good friends Break from home People talk to you Meals taken care of Activities to do	24-hour care Staff input	Medication
Negative	Not very clean	Lack of staff	Treatment unclear
	Violent patients	Violent staff	Side-effects
	Institutionalization	Inefficient staff	
	Drug dealing	Lack of support	
	Possessions stolen	Lack of interaction	
	Lack of activities	Lack of qualified/ knowledgeable staff	
	Confined to ward	Lack of sensitivity/caring	
	Lack of privacy	Losing user possessions	
	Visitors upset by ward		

* Each user can appear in more than one category.

variable and on the whole not good.' 'Very variable' is a good way of summarizing user attitudes and experiences of hospital care. Patrick, for instance, comments,

> I must have picked a particularly good time, because normally it's like a hell hole if you go to a psychiatric unit. You know, you've all the dizzies about. People are just totally not there. I picked the right 12 weeks because everyone who was there were quite a good crew, you know. I right enjoyed it, the food was marvelous, the people were marvelous, the staff were marvelous.

Positive aspects of hospital tended to surround the social situation that users found themselves in. Thus, meeting other people and making new friends was a real plus for many, even if the treatment on the whole had been disappointing. Hospital also offered a form of escape or 'break' from the outside world and particular troubles at home, as Duncan notes,

> Yeah, I were fine in hospital. That's why sometimes I ask if I can... have a break like, you know, 'cos of the voices and that, you

> know, if I get out of the way, get out of the house and get out of the way of them. It's as though they're in the house talking... like you're talking to me.

There were also personal economic advantages to being under hospital care: heating, accommodation, activities and food are all free. As Alan explains,

> [The hospital staff] tret me great, you know, food were great, like I say, them pills what they give you, were... really helped me, so I just sat in there, watching TV, getting fat, you know. It were good... I think everybody needs a holiday like that.

Receiving treatment at hospital, or facilitating recovery from a trauma, seems to become secondary for many users. This situation is summed up by Roger in answer to my question 'so, the hospital works for you?': 'well, in the respect that I eventually get better, and come out, I suppose you can say... it's worked, I don't know... I don't know how else you could look at the problem really.' The very discharge of a mental health user from hospital becomes the benchmark of success for institutional psychiatry.

6.4.2 Staff

From the user narratives we find a general picture of staff apathy on the wards. Good, 'caring' staff are the exception. For instance Sheila states, 'there were some super staff, they really were, and they cared'. In this case, staff would bring 'cream cakes an' all sorts for supper, there were lots to do – they organized music quizzes and you could go and play table tennis'. Yet more often users can point to the many incidents where staff have been unhelpful or inefficient. For example, Anita comments,

> The majority of staff have always been... quite unfriendly, quite unhelpful. This is with the exception of, you know, an odd few who were really nice... I've been in five times now and I've always found staff to be a problem. A lot of them are not approachable. I've been in some very, very distressed situations and just been ignored, completely ignored.

The psychiatrist responsible for consultation and management of the user's treatment would often change, leading to a lack of consistency and meaning that users would often have to repeat their illness history for each new psychiatrist. Consultants were also generally difficult to get hold of. Despite these factors, most users were sympathetic to the lack of time the consultants had available for individual cases, and generally felt they were dealt with in a decent manner (usually due to either getting the 'right medication' or feeling that the consultant had understood their problems). David makes a statement typical of many:

> [The consultant] was quite sympathetic and sorted my medication out quite well... and he was sound, seemed to know, you know what he was doing and he, he were great, but it was just the, the day-to-day, 24-hour care on the ward was pathetic.

The lack of contact between nurses and users is further illustrated by David, who was himself a nurse at another hospital. He points out the potential dangers of the staff neglecting contact with users:

> When I came to discharge... the nurse who was my primary nurse, he was, like, most involved in my case, who should know everything that was going on... in a position of having someone with my history asking to discharge themselves should be very careful and ask them some very pertinent questions, and decide whether (a) he's gonna hold me or (b) he's gonna let me go. And... his pertinent question was 'you don't want to go because of those thoughts in your head do you?' Which, like, was a pretty naff question. And I said 'no'. You know, 'oh, it's all right then, off you go'... He's just let me through those doors without any formal assessment at all, quite dangerously to himself.

Many times these user narratives recount a lack of contact or interest in them from any of the hospital staff. Shakila states,

> I thought [the hospital staff] wasn't giving us much help... like, you know, we were admitted and they were just coming to regular check-ups after each hour or whatever when they had to. And they weren't really bothered... they didn't really... physically, like looking at a person. They didn't used to give us advice what we need to do. Like if we needed something, they wouldn't be there.

In Jai's case this becomes quite concerning:

> [The hospital staff] never really counselled me and...the service that they were providing wasn't that good as well. And from the very first time I went in, when I was stiff and that, I had problems going to the toilet and nobody would help me.

One of the hospital ward's concept of '24-hour care' was outlined by another user:

> Oh yeah, they were supposed to be there on duty for any people that woke up in the night and needed something. There were a few patients that specifically got up in the night and started screaming their heads off through some illness, and other occasions the night staff, they were asleep. I got up to go to the toilet and they were asleep, sat in these types and chairs and they're there, fast asleep. So I, I asked about that, I said, 'how come the night staff are asleep?' They said, 'well they've nothing to do on a night, what do you expect them to do?' I said, 'I expect them to be awake in case there's some emergency'. I couldn't believe that – they were fast asleep, mainly the ladies, and they were more or less the same staff on all night, because of doing nights probably, 'cos they were easier rather than the day shift. But I couldn't believe it when they were asleep.

In some cases, it appears as if the staff simply hoped the users would leave the hospital of their own accord, as happened in David's case:

> I was there for a week, but not a single member of staff came and talked to me or found out what was going on... There's other... little things that they were doing that I wasn't liking so, I signed myself out.

The 'other things' he mentioned included being expected to have his diabetes injection (administered to his bottom) in view of the rest of the staff and users on the ward.

These narratives beg the question as to what functions the hospital staff actually serve; these appear to be limited to either administrative or policing functions on the ward. Lack of staffing is sometimes mentioned by users – who have some sympathy with the current situation – but a question remains as to how experiences can be so different from one ward to another if the staffing situation is similar across the whole psychiatric hospital. There is little doubt from the narratives that at least some of the staff do not fundamentally 'care' about the users. This is reflected in comments from the narratives which mention such things as staff 'looking down' on users, being unsympathetic when the users have been in (physical as well as emotional) pain, and even being violent towards users. The latter complaint is expressed in the following quote from a man with a Pakistani background who explains how he saw one user on the ward punching an old Asian woman (also a user). He retaliated in turn by kicking her attacker;

> And [the ward staff] seen me kicking him and then they came running, and they grabbed me and they pinned me down and I couldn't breathe for about a couple of minutes. I go 'let me go', you know, I was shouting really loud and my cousin, my cousin, brother was there and my little brother was there as well, and my other cousin, brother, and they go 'let him go', you know, and they told them to go, to leave the hospital, and they had to go and they let me go then, yeah, but whilst they wouldn't let me go, you know, I was, and then I couldn't breathe, and this and that, and they go 'well you were violent'.

Though there were some sensitive and helpful nurses who would sit and talk with users, many others were more likely to avoid such contact. Even when staff did have to interact with users this could be done in a derogatory manner, with Anita remembering that her visiting sister was horrified 'over the way staff have spoken to the patients, as if they're scum really'. She cites one incidence as an example:

> When it's medication time they'll [staff] shout in wherever you're sat, they'll shout in 'tablets', you know, and you've to queue up for your tablets in a big row. And one of the patients in there had said, she'd said to him something like 'Johnny, are you coming for your tablets?' And he said, 'no I'm not', but, I mean, three quarters of the patients refused their tablets anyway and they've got to be gently coaxed a lot of them. Some of them refuse point blank. They can't do anything about it but this particular nurse just said 'oh suit yourself then'. She didn't try and coax him or anything. Then he had some sort of an attack, whatever, and he's asking for his tablets, and she refused completely to give him 'em. She said 'he refused them, he won't', and this is probably only three quarters of an hour afterwards he'd refused, he'd refused them so she weren't prepared to go an' open the trolley and give him 'em. So, there's all sorts of things like that going on.

It was luck of the draw whether users found a more caring and sympathetic member of staff when they were in hospital, though many said they would have liked the staff to take at least a few minutes of their time to talk to them.

6.4.3 Treatment

As medical staff are left with mainly administrative or policing roles on the ward, 'treatment' is left to what the psychiatrist in charge prescribes – normally medication and, in a few cases, ECT. Some users expected more than just this:

> I wasn't getting any treatment in [the psychiatric hospital] anyway. I was getting medication and that was it. There was nothing else going on, and I can do that myself at home, you know – go to my GP and get exactly the same drugs and do it myself. (David)

> The treatment? What sort of treatment? They don't give me any treatment, all they give is medication. (Jai)

Many of the user narratives, however, do express the usefulness of the drug treatment in 'stabilizing' their condition or helping their recovery. At the same time there is a concern that not enough information is given – by the consultants – about the possible side-effects and dangers of taking such medication long-term. A number of narratives illustrate this point:

> [I] started taking more tablets and more tablets, they were making me poorly, like, you know, and anyway they've taken me off 'em now. I don't take 'em at all now, like, but I've no effects for wanting 'em, you know, but when I were, when I had 'em I were wanting 'em all the time like drugs. (Duncan)

> I'm on tablets now and I hate it, because I want to be normal, I don't want to have to take tablets. I was on Lithium [a mood stabilizer often used in cases of manic depression and recurring depression]... I hated it... I kept going back to doctors and saying 'I want to come off this Lithium', and 'oh no... you've gotta be on it for five years', and I went and read up about Lithium. The more I read about it the more I wanted to be off it. (Helen)

> [The medication] don't do anything to me, I mean I don't feel any effect off them. But they must be, I presume they must be doing

> something, 'cos I am a lot calmer... It's just I'm so used to pill poppin' that... you know, you could stuff anything down ma throat and I probably wouldn't notice... you get to that point. (Tracy)

The issue of using psychotropic medication as a normal part of psychiatric treatment has been critiqued elsewhere (see for instance, Bracken and Thomas 2001; Breggin 1993). Suffice to say here that a quarter of the narratives were fully negative about this treatment, with the spectre of unpleasant side-effects being mentioned by most of the users on medication. At its most extreme the medication *caused* a total breakdown, but more often the complaints were of drowsiness, tiredness, stomach pains, shaking, weight gain, lock-jaw, and mouth and nose feeling dry and 'woolly'. More permanent damage was suggested by a number of users who cited liver and kidney complaints. In some cases, users talked of not being able to perform even the simplest of tasks whilst on high dosages of medication (for a good overview of psychotropic medication and possible side effects, see MIND 2007b).

The controversial treatment of ECT was given to at least eight of the users in the research. Most were happy with the treatment to the extent that it appeared to 'calm' or 'cure' the illness (in particular, the hearing of voices), though for some this turned out to be only temporary. Anita explains,

> The ECT... I felt... after probably a week when I'd finished the last, had the last one, I thought it was a miraculous cure. I felt like a different person. I thought this is it, they've cured me. And that lasted, that feeling lasted for four weeks, and then I went into a severe depression. So it didn't work.

A good analogy was made at a mental health conference I attended whilst carrying out the fieldwork. A user commented that ECT works in the same way as when a television is not working properly and you hit it a few times until it has a clear picture again. You do not know why it is working again – it may, indeed, be damaged inside – but for now it is alright. It is still true that psychiatry has no real idea what ECT actually does to a person. The remark that is often made in its defence is that 'it seems to work'. Some users still ask for ECT and they feel it works for them, but nevertheless side-effects are reported. The most frequent side-effect for ECT noted in the narratives was memory loss. Pro-ECT psychiatry argues that this is only short-term memory loss, but as Anita put it, 'me concentration levels are really poor and it's two years since I had the ECT now, and it's really affected ma memory'. Bill, an artist, comments on the ECT he had a number of years ago: 'I'm not too bad at memory recall at the moment, but names sometimes escape me, artists I've worked with, you know, and the like.' On the other hand, Duncan is positive about ECT. He says it was 'to help me forget like, you know, what I'd been going through'. Maybe a treatment which offers the chance to forget can also be useful for some users?

6.4.4 Improvements

Many of the improvements expressed within the user narratives centred on the ward staff's need to interact more with users. Nurses should be more sensitive and patient with users, be able to empathize, listen and offer advice to users. Nurses – especially assigned 'key workers' – should make a point of being available for consultations and to deal with the difficulties users experience. In turn, there was a need for the ward staff to be better trained in mental health issues, to have knowledge of different user problems and situations (self-harm was one example cited), to be more efficient in their approach to ward organization, and generally to be more positive and affable. Lesley sums up a number of the issues here:

> I don't expect the staff to be sat there with a cup of coffee and a newspaper... [in] the lounge area where everybody sits. They could be talking to people. I reported one for that, when I was very down and needed somebody to talk to. But of course I didn't get anywhere, these reports... you'll get nowhere. There's no point in having a complaint or a compliment box on that board, 'cos you don't win, never.... If they've got spare time they should be out talking to the patients... I think the patients help each other rather than the staff helping the patients. And, like, new people that have just arrived there, some of them are so doped they can just say something, like mutter 'water', they want some water and it's always the patients that go get them the water, the staff just ignore them until they're interviewed by the doctor. Which is disgusting, they should keep an eye on them. Like all I had on were my dressing gown when I first went in there, yeah, and eventually it was a patient that asked if I could have a blanket or something to wrap 'round me as well, with there being men and women walking in and out. 'Cos they'd put me in like the view of the door, the main door, so anybody could have been in and out, and I was sat there for going on four hours before I was interviewed by a doctor. And my husband didn't know where I was or anything. I asked them to phone his work but he never got a message. It was Sunday and he worked two 'till four, and he never got the message.

Users were also concerned about the lack of control of dangerous patients. A number of people generally felt unsafe in a place they were hoping would offer some sanctuary. There was also a felt need for more privacy, especially for consultations with staff and when users received visitors. Sometimes there appeared to be little or 'nothing to do' in hospital. This sense of apathy permeates the narratives. Thus, users suggested more activities and being able to go outside the hospital to be involved in local organized activities. Further, some suggested they could have benefited from some formal counselling or psychotherapy whilst hospitalized. Generally, users were concerned at the feeling of organized chaos that was experienced on many of the wards. If there was an infrastructure, the users did not see or recognize one whilst they were there.

6.5 Bradford Home Treatment Service

Given the user narratives on hospitalization it was always likely that treatment at home was going to be considered better. But what actually does the treatment consist of and is it really so different – practically rather than philosophically – to hospital care? Is it only being

Table 6.3 Positive and negative aspects of home treatment summarized from the user narratives*

Positive	Staff who listen, talk and are supportive	12
	Being in my own environment	7
	Having one-to-one input	6
	Being able to phone staff/have mobile phone	6
	Dealing with my medication	5
	Helping my family/partner	4
	Helping me practise relaxation techniques	4
	The flexibility and time staff have for me	4
	Helping me get out more	3
	Having trust and respect for me	3
	Staff emphasizing positive thinking for me	3
	Offering me advice and information	2
	Having ethnic minority/bilingual staff	1
Negative	Too short a period of time	3
	Too forceful and domineering	3
	Emphasis on medication	2
	Promised things not delivered	1
	They hospitalized me	1

* Each user can appear in more than one category.

at home that makes users feel better about the service or does it have anything to do with the quality of care? From content analysis of the 20 home treatment user narratives, Table 6.3 shows a list of the major positive and negative points from their experiences of home treatment.

Given the earlier comments about what users felt they needed and were not getting from the hospital system, it is unsurprising that when home treatment have met these needs there has been much praise for them. Often a combination of factors were felt to have improved their quality of life, such as receiving one-to-one staff input, being 'treated' in their own environment and being encouraged to get out of the house more. Some examples of these positive narratives are given below:

> I found it [the BHTS] very useful... because it was an alternative to hospital and it meant that I could actually get treatment here [at home], plus there was someone coming in every day. You see what I mean, 'cos I were really desperate at the time, really bad, you know, with my nerves and that, so it helped, you know, with somebody coming in. Just somebody being there, plus knowing they were a phone call away when they wasn't here... so we had like night-cover as well. (Suzie)

> For me, it was being able to talk things over with someone, and somebody to sort of turn the negative things round that you were thinking and get you to think positively about them, because I realized I was dwelling too much on the negatives and they [the BHTS] were able to say 'well, yes, I can appreciate that, you know, that's how you feel but...' And sort of putting 'buts' in, were able to make me think more positive and they also were able to teach me relaxation techniques that I've been able to use quite effectively just lately. To listening to tapes and relaxing when I've felt all wound up. So that's been very useful. (Tony)

> [The BHTS] were willing to come out every day, spend hours. Whereas others had tight appointments, they had appointments but they worked an agenda out and they'd spend two hours, three hours with me. On one occasion they'd take me out for a walk here and there, to get some fresh air and the rest of it when I first met [BHTS staff member]. So I mean that built me confidence, helped me trust and the rest of it. (Liam)

As well as the intensive staff input received, users praised the help given to their families in helping them cope with the crisis. Further, the narratives note home treatment staff dealing with factors such as their medication. After consultation with the users, medication could be changed and reduced (see also Bracken and Cohen 1999). There is a sense of flexibility and sensitivity in staff dealing with users in their own homes and this leads a number of users to talk of substantial improvements in their quality of life. Michael, for instance, comments,

> [Psychiatric hospital] didn't actually help me long-term, but it helped me at the time. Whereas home treatment has helped me long-term, I feel. It's given me a lot firmer understanding of all my problems and how to deal with my problems and go about my life.

Liam adds that 'the hospital bit you can miss out completely. I couldn't have developed. But as a better person, from that home treatment service, yeah, it helped me develop'.

Some users, however, found there to be problems with the home treatment service, such as some staff members spending little time with them, being too forceful in their approach and relying more on medication. In one case, activities were promised but not delivered. Samples of narratives illustrating these points are given below:

> Well, I didn't think they [the BHTS] understood fully, because they didn't come in long enough. If they had come in long enough, I could have got a lot more off my chest, see, with them, which I wanted to do... but I didn't get that. So then I ended up... at the beginning again. I just, I did the same thing again and I feel that if they'd have come in long enough, I wouldn't have [got] to that position again with it.... But there were relaxation that they did teach me how to use, and then there was talking about taking me swimming and taking me for a sauna, but it never come to that, 'cos they didn't come long enough. (Garth)

> [The BHTS staff] don't stay long... for a few minutes... between five and 15 at the most. I think it's with them not knowing you, they should stop and talk to you. In hospital they do sometimes, but not the last time I was in... [The BHTS staff] just bring the tablets mainly, and a bit a talking when [BHTS staff member] was here. (Celia)

> [The BHTS psychiatrist] it was that advised me not to go into hospital, was obviously a very learned man, and he knows his job and he

> knows what he's talking about, so then I felt pressurized to accept his point of view, you see. And, which I did on three occasions, and each time they'd gone away and I'd left it a week, I went so downhill again, and I'd been going crazy in the house and I'd feel like I'd been abandoned in that instance really. (Michael)

Fifteen out of the 20 home treatment user narratives indicated that home treatment had been a better option than hospital. Whereas only two users stated that home treatment was less favourable than hospital. Similar positive findings appear in other studies that measure home treatment and hospital care in more quantitative formats (for example, Bracken and Cohen 1999; Fenton *et al.* 1979, 1984; Hoult *et al.* 1983; Muijen *et al.* 1992; Orme and Cohen 2001; Smyth and Hoult 2000; Test and Stein 1980). Given the inadequacies of hospital treatment we have noted, community alternatives like home treatment are obviously more likely to achieve positive outcomes for users and their families.

A varied range of improvements were suggested for home treatment. The service itself occasionally 'cut off' users too soon, staff time was limited and sometimes there was a need for more activities or further counselling with the user. The feeling of the treatment being 'user-centred' did not apply in at least a number of cases, as the service took decisions to minimize contact and resources available without user consent. Further resources for home treatment were also suggested, such as a 'halfway house' so as to avoid hospitalization if having problems at home, having sites other than the psychiatric hospital in which to meet other people socially, increasing the number of staff on the home treatment service (so as to spend more time with users) and having comprehensive care plans to deal with the transfer of users from the BHTS to the local community mental health resource teams.

6.6 Conclusion

Precipitating factors to a crisis requiring psychiatric intervention were mostly self-defined by users as socially caused. The referral system into hospital or on to home treatment remained something of a lottery here. Experiences of hospitalization were varied with the general care being negligible. Ward staff were heavily criticized by many of the users, and 'treatment' was defined largely as medication and ECT. Despite hospital still being perceived as a significant part of 'the balanced system of care' (Thornicroft and Tansella 2004), it appears from the narratives that insufficient thought is given to treatment options within the institution.

As community options continue to expand, it is important that medical professionals and policy makers do not neglect reviews of in-patient provision.

Unsurprisingly, the BHTS was found to be a better form of psychiatric care than hospitalization for many. Improved quality of care was found in terms of staff, treatment and being at home. Significantly, treatment options that went beyond medication and ECT were facilitated by the BHTS. Interventions with users included relaxation techniques and exercise as well as social interventions such as shopping trips and offering support to carers. Above all, the narratives cited the helpfulness of one-to-one interactions and active input from the BHTS staff. Nevertheless, there was also room for improvement at the home treatment service, with staff sometimes being overbearing and making unfulfilled promises to users.

There was a perceived problem of the continuity of care between different parts of the local mental health care system: whether the user was at hospital or with the BHTS there was not a feeling of common ownership of an individual's problems. Thus, users often felt their histories were not understood by the different groups of staff, that staff turnover and changeover led to confusion and disruption as to the user's current status (which often led to misdiagnosis as well) and that there was a lack of communication between different parts of the system (one user mentioned that at least with home treatment, the different staff they dealt with seemed to know their case history). The feeling of chaos on the ward is partly replicated by the wider system of local mental health care, which is anything but 'seamless' (see Cohen 1997b, 1999a; Ledwith *et al.* 1997). Without this important fault being rectified, users will continue to suffer bad practice to a lesser or greater extent in whichever service they are attached to. In both cases, reference was made to involvement of ex-users in their treatment in some capacity. Tied to this was a lack of knowledge about user-related groups (such as the Hearing Voices Network, which has a local group not far from Bradford). This suggests a need to look further at user involvement in the development of services in more than a tokenistic way. Appropriately then, in Chapter 7 user accounts of recovery and their own coping techniques will be explored.

7
Recovery from Illness and Self-Coping

> Even though I couldn't go into town, I used to force myself to go to town. You sort of like throw yourself in the deep end. I thought, 'well, if I get a taxi, end up in town, get out of the taxi, then there's nothing I can do – I'm in town, so I'll have to face it'. I've always been like that you know, pushy you know, trying to push myself forward.
>
> (Tony)

7.1 Summary

Chapter 6 surveyed the descent into illness and psychiatric interventions experienced by the users. It was shown that a variety of socially focused factors are usually involved in bringing about a crisis, yet treatment is biomedically orientated towards a control of symptoms. But how do users explain their illness experiences themselves? This chapter explores further illness meanings from the narratives collected. It will be demonstrated that users can develop different understandings of their crises depending on the psychiatric treatment received. The narratives will also demonstrate a range of self-coping techniques that promote recovery and well-being, in turn, offering the hope of a future without biomedical treatment and further psychiatric intervention.

7.2 Current state of being

There are general – if sometimes overlapping – differences in current states of being between clusters of users which I have called the 'unwell', those 'getting by' and those who are 'well'. As far as possible these are self-defined by the users. It does not refer to a stage of their supposed psychiatric illness but rather a 'state of being' within their total life experience (whether work, relationships, leisure, illness or whatever). These groups are described below.

7.2.1 The 'unwell'

Patrick's narrative is one which emphasizes a kind of melancholy and sadness which appears to engulf his life. 'Look at me,' he says, 'I'm at the wrong side of sixty but I still, it still doesn't depress me in that respect. I thought "I've had my life and that's it".' His life encompasses over 30 years of psychiatric hospitals and treatment, as well as 15 years in the marines which he joined when he was 15 years old. Apart from talking about his time serving in Korea and the Middle East, he mentions the strict discipline he experienced in the marines:

> They built this new depot down in Deal in Kent. And we were on the parade this morning, we had this old DI, you know, drill instructor. And he come from the old school, you know. He'd joined up about 1930 or something. He says, 'now', he says, 'I'm gonna show you some discipline'. He says, 'I'll pick any squad,' he says, 'I'm gonna pick 672 squad'. He said, 'second from the first rank, pace forward'. So this was the squad behind me. So this junior marine steps forward, he says, 'turn left, double to the wall and bang your head against it 'til it bleeds'. And I'm not joking. And the kid done it, he went bong, bong, bong. There were blood all over the place. That was the sort of thing in them days. You see nowadays, this is why, I know you can't compare A to B, and the sort of thing that sticks in my craw because it's there at the back of my mind all the time.

After being raised in an orphanage and serving in the marines, Patrick found decent employment and bought himself a house. He married soon afterwards and had two children. As he says, 'we had everything going for us, but it just seemed to, seemed to get to my head. I don't know why but it did. I couldn't cope with it'. Despite continuing his work, he began to drink heavily and experienced his first periods of hospitalization. He shows me some of his scars from suicide attempts. His wife later died of cancer. Patrick tells me he gets bad asthma attacks which results in mobility problems, though he has some friends who visit him regularly.

Presenting these segments from Patrick's narrative is not to show that all users are 'victims' or 'sad characters', but rather to show that some of the narratives outline certain similar characteristics, in the case of the 'unwell' it is often loneliness, melancholy and long periods of reflection on the past. These narratives are full of the negative aspects of a person's life. For instance, Duncan – who is a similar age to Patrick and has also had many years in hospital – talks of the pain and sadness of his parents dying and how lonely life is without them. There is also a certain fatalism within these user narratives, an acceptance of future relapse and the need for psychiatric treatment; psychiatry is a regular part of their lives.

7.2.2 Getting by

In contrast to those who fall into the 'unwell' category, those who are 'getting by' are usually attempting some conscious effort to 'get well' and 'not be poorly'. There are, however, barriers and issues to face that mean this will take time and further support, or recognition and facilitation of certain conditions. The majority of the narratives fall into this category.

As examples of those 'getting by', we find barriers such as being able to get a job, being able to get out of the house or having physical illnesses that restrict health and well-being. Many of these problems are reflected in Gillian's narrative; she finds it difficult to leave her house because of the possibility of panic attacks. She would like to study and get a job, and is very bored with being stuck at home (as well as the economic hardships of this). She cannot, however, predict when she will have an attack and this restricts her ability to take college courses or work outside the home. Additionally, the support of a CPN was withdrawn from her because she disagreed with the (medical) treatment she received.

The people who are 'getting by' have some determination that they do not want to go back to psychiatric hospital or forever be reliant on psychiatric care. They want to be 'better' and live the so-called 'normal life'. Though they have barriers to progress – and some believe they will occasionally need hospital again – there is more resolve to live and to get through bad times. Whereas the 'unwell' accept the illness as part of them, those who are 'getting by' see it more as a period of time that could be behind them. They usually know what they need to help them progress, for example, one-to-one supervision and counselling, encouragement to get out and do things, flexible learning, training and employment provision, child care and so on. There is a real sense that this group are fighting if not always winning in their lives. These people were found to be often younger in age and female. Possible reasons for this may be because these people have had less years of psychiatry or are experiencing newly found independence from others (particularly in the case of those women who experienced a period of crisis due to divorce or separation).

7.2.3 The 'well'

Unlike the other two groups, 'the well' see the period of distress/illness in the past. Whether they have a perceived explanation for what happened to them (or what was done to them) or not, the events of being ill or being under psychiatric care are already behind them. The crisis was a 'freak occurrence' in their lives and has little meaning for them now. This group is more likely to talk of the future and of other factors which seem to have no connection to their illness (for example, Rachel's narrative in Section 5.4).

This short separation of the users into three groups is to illustrate that different 'types' of narratives were encountered by the author. It appears that there may be differences in perceptions of illness state between social classes, gender groups, ethnic minority groups and different generations of user. This is not to suggest that there is any 'right' or 'wrong' way to understand and conceptualize life experiences and illness and health within them; it is more to help the reader understand different life perceptions. Psychiatry talks of people who 'engage' with their illness and with treatment as if this is something necessary before recovery can happen. In outlining these groups it will become clearer that 'engagement' is not necessary for a sense of well-being. People can perceive themselves as 'well' without awareness or understanding of their illness, or as more or less permanently 'unwell' and be very aware of what their illness means to them.

7.3 The meaning of illness

Although all the users in this research were diagnosed with a 'severe mental illness' and, therefore, would have received a psychotic label to explain their behaviour, the narratives show that users actually self-define their illness in a variety of ways. Nevertheless, psychiatric diagnoses were used by some to explain their trauma. For example, the 'psychotic' labels of 'manic depression' and 'schizophrenia' were commonly used by the group that had experienced only psychiatric hospital. In contrast, those who had experienced the BHTS were more

Table 7.1 Self-definitions of user illness extracted from the user narratives*

	Hospital	Home treatment	Total
Manic depression	6	0	6
Schizophrenia	2	1	3
Hearing voices	3	1	4
Depression	2	7	9
Attempted suicide	3	0	3
Paranoia	0	2	2
Alcohol or drug mental illness	3	0	3
Other	6	6	12
Total	25	17	42

* Each user has been assigned to one category only.

likely to use the term 'depression', and this term becomes almost generic for how the users describe their suffering. A full list of self-definitions from the narratives (where people stated them) is given in Table 7.1.

The most obvious conclusion that can be drawn from the observations in Table 7.1 is that the hospital group were a more 'severe' group than those interviewed from the BHTS (that is, the hospital sample included more people who defined their illness as either 'manic depression' or 'schizophrenia'). However, quantitative research evidence has shown that both treatment options dealt with similar client groups (see Bracken and Cohen 1999; Cohen 1999a), and the research in this book has sought to match appropriately (see Chapter 4). The analysis suggests, then, that there may be a more fundamental reason for the different self-definitions of illness.

It must be stressed that all the definitions of psychopathologies and so on are the user's own taken from their personal narratives. Many users gave detailed insights into their illnesses and, subsequently, a difference appeared in the understanding of their lives depending on the psychiatric treatment option received. For example, those who may have felt themselves to be 'psychotic' previous to home treatment's input, were more likely, post-home treatment, to suggest 'bad feelings' and 'depression' were root factors for them now. The illness was not always behind them – a number were worried about, or even expected, 'relapse' – but there was a positive attitude towards the possibility of *change* and of moving forward. There was generally less optimism within the hospital group, with a reliance on psychotic labels and medication to 'control' or 'level' their symptoms. Here are a couple of quotations which illustrate this difference, the first from a hospital user, the second from a home treatment user;

> When I read the pamphlet in the hospital about... aspects of schizophrenia and it did relate to me personal experience, you know – people talking about me in the background, discussing, things like that, you know... I don't think I'm a lot different from a lot of me friends who I know were schizophrenic... I mean I've had these voices for, what, 31 years altogether. I mean there just something I put up with, you know. (James)

> It was more of a depression, the state that I was in, it wasn't more of a manic depression or anything of that nature. It was just acute depression.... My illness was an isolated illness, as I didn't come across anyone who was suffering from what I was suffering from [in psychiatric hospital]. (Yunas)

There was wide variation in the two groups of narratives but, generally, they follow the pattern indicated here. This result also suggests that in *all* cases the psychiatric narrative appears to have superseded users' own narratives. In the hospital-only narratives the emphasis is placed on the dominant medical model of diagnosis and treatment, at home treatment there is a more liberal view which seeks to avoid such diagnoses and aims to deal with life factors instead. In both cases the user narratives are subsumed under a different psychiatric narrative. The concern is that both psychiatric narratives disrupt a cohesive inner meaning for periods of crises.

It might appear obvious that the user narratives will differ given the ability of psychiatric professionals to influence the life stories of users. The pessimism of a fixed medical model given to users in hospital is likely to change with a group of medical professionals who take a different model of care and come to the user's home (a place which appears to have a central point in many users' existence and problems related to their illness). Nevertheless, it remains a significant finding. The narratives have shown that mental health user perceptions of their circumstances and illness can *change*, rather than being static. If medical professionals choose to strike the psychotic labels from their treatment, then psychoses can no longer create the life sentences seen in some of the narratives (especially for the 'unwell' group of users). This can be demonstrated further with a couple of short examples below (firstly a hospital user, then a home treatment user).

Roger has been a teacher and photographer, he says his illness is 'chemically based' – that is what the psychiatrist has said. He is 'either being high or low...the label is manic depression, so I've been at one end of the scale or the other'. He says he would like to try other therapies if they were available, rather than only relying on the medication. He also comments that he could do with 'a complete change', feels this might do him good, because 'I'm just stagnating here, nothing's happening at all'.

Paul has had mood swings similar to Roger's. He has been self-employed in a number of different capacities including car selling. He says of his illness,

> Basically I just experiment with myself...I know it's crazy and stupid...I went out of control, I couldn't control myself and so I've gone into areas of me mind where perhaps I shouldn't have delved 'cos I opened doors to insanity.

Further, he emphasizes his own definition of his illness:

> Mine were a nice kind of insanity, my depression just means that I have mood swings and everybody has mood swings. I've said this to you before, you get up in a morning and you feel shit but a couple of hours later, put some music on, relax, your mood come round where it's really, really loving and you want some female company, you know.

Whereas hospital users were still struggling to make sense of their lives and their illness, the BHTS users were attempting to move forward. Particularly when those who heard voices (this group is considered 'psychotic' in the ICD and DSM classifications) were considered, there were sizeable differences between the hospital and home treatment groups. There appears to be a relationship between being lonely, on your own and/or family bereavement that makes it more likely that hearing voices will occur. A couple of examples from the narratives of people who hear voices are shown below (the first, a hospital user, the second, a BHTS user). It will be seen that whereas the hospital user still feels 'in the middle' of his illness, the home treatment user is talking in the past tense:

> You see, all these voices are talking, it's spoiling me mind...I'm thinking what they're saying, like, you know, whereas in hospital if

> somebody talks to me I think what they say, like, you know, and I talk back to 'em...I can ignore them in hospital. I don't hear 'em in hospital, it's truth, honest I don't. Just when I sit in me loneliness you know. (Duncan)

> I didn't step a foot outside the house and I was very paranoid, thinking that people had heard that I wasn't going out of the house and were talking about me, whispering behind my back, saying 'this is what you get'...and, like, voices in my head kind of thing of thing, almost like whispering. I thought they were talking about me and that didn't help matters. (Raiza)

It is interesting that many of the issues that affect people through their illness surround their relationship to their home, whether it be family, mobility or spatial factors. Hospital, to a limited degree, has helped users cope outside the home (or to 'get away' from the home). Unfortunately, the problems are then transferred to the unreal world of the psychiatric hospital. Treatment of users in their home environment would appear to encourage more positive, long-term outcomes for many.

7.4 Self-coping strategies

One wonders how users cope without calling on further psychiatric treatment. Particularly if the user is in dispute with the treatment he or she receives, how does the user react in a future crisis? How do they help themselves? Maybe through knowing more about users' self-coping techniques we can learn something fundamental about the nature of different periods of crisis and illness. Further content analysis of the narratives illustrates a wide variety of practices which users see as facilitating coping with their illness on a day-to-day level (other than medication, which many were still taking). It should be noted that the activities mentioned were emphasized as 'therapeutic' in the user narratives, not just hobbies or interests. From Table 7.2 we can see the important therapeutic value of users interacting with others, not just through socializing with others or being involved in college courses and so on, but also through working, of which Claudette comments, 'now I'm working in a supermarket. And there's lots of people. I'm meeting people every day...and I'm really enjoying it...I go out more now'. Time and again it was stated that work was not simply an economic necessity but had important social implications in users feeling wanted, integrated and belonging to society rather feeling outside of it.

Table 7.2 Self-coping techniques extracted from user narratives*

	Hospital	Home treatment	Total
Socializing with friends/family	3	5	8
Sleeping	4	2	6
Other	3	2	5
Music	3	1	4
Painting/drawing	2	2	4
Walking	2	2	4
Work	2	2	4
Alternative therapies	1	2	3
Exercise	1	2	3
Going out	1	2	3
Relaxation techniques	0	3	3
Alcohol	1	1	2
College courses	1	1	2
Illegal drugs	2	0	2
Having a child to care for	0	2	2
Housework/looking after home	1	1	2
Pets	0	2	2
Shopping	1	1	2
Poetry	0	1	1
Religious practices	0	1	1
Watching television	1	0	1

* Each user can appear in more than one category.

The problem of being at home and having time on one's hands was overcome for some by 'getting out', shopping, walking, driving and so on. For those who had difficulties leaving their house, there was also therapeutic value gained from taking up arts, playing or listening to music, watching television, looking after the house or simply 'stroking the dog' as in one case. Drinking alcohol and taking (illegal) drugs were also therapeutic for some in acting as a relaxant or stimulant. As Gillian remarks,

> I used to smoke cannabis... that really did help but I can't afford it now... It seems to open your mind 'n' all, I don't know... that's just my imagination but it does. I usually think better. You have all these mad ideas (laughs).

In some cases, drugs or alcohol have helped confidence and allowed users who were usually house-bound to have a night out with their friends. There is a strong possibility that home treatment psychiatry has encouraged people to take up self-coping mechanisms as, generally, this group of users mentioned more self-coping strategies than those who had only experienced hospital treatment. This includes the references made to relaxation techniques and alternative therapies as ways of self-coping. One user specifically pointed to home treatment's help in facilitating her search for alternative remedies such as aromatherapy oils and acupuncture, with the long-term hope that these would replace the large amount of medication she was taking. There are a couple more self-coping strategies to briefly draw the reader's attention to. One is the value of sleep to users. This might be seen as quite a negative way of coping with one's illness but the narratives expressed the healing qualities of the process: it was described as 'a release' by Zed, and Dylan stated, similarly,

> I feel better when I'm asleep, I feel alright when I'm in a different dimension, I'm free when sleeping, not dealing with all the stress, problem is you can only stay in bed for so long, then you can't sleep anymore.

Another interesting issue that arose was the therapeutic power of having a baby or raising a child for female users. Having a child was a reason to 'stay well', there was more at stake than the user's own health and a feeling of 'duty' towards their dependants. As one user explained, 'if it wasn't for the children, I think I'd have gone completely off my rocker... I know that I have to keep part of my head together, I know I have to'.

7.5 Spiritualism

As we have seen, there are many different ways in which users can perceive and understand their own periods of illness, as well as how they react and cope with these crises. Although religious and spiritual practices were not often cited by users as a healing practice, it nevertheless had particular significance for some. There was a marked divide between white and ethnic minority users here, with only five white user narratives (all male) containing reference to particular beliefs, whereas eight ethnic minority users mentioned some spiritual elements. The differences in personal meaning were also highlighted.

White users talked of their faith in God, or somebody 'up there' and Christianity. One user went so far as to say that he was not one for talking to psychiatrists but preferred to talk to 'him' (God) instead. One user believed he was Jesus Christ, another that he had seen Jesus

Christ. In the latter case, the user had told his psychiatrist about this and was disappointed when this was dismissed as impossible (indeed these narratives are typically seen by psychiatrists as a further symptom of the user's mental illness, see for example Susko 1994; Szasz 1971). The user commented on the reason why he saw Jesus and continues to hear spirits and voices: 'you lose somebody and somebody comes back,' he explained. Duncan's mother and grandmother were both dead and he admitted that their deaths had deeply affected him. He sees the voices as part of an 'afterlife', the dead coming back. He also had a friend who had died recently and believes that his spirit had returned, not just through the voices but by generally living in the material world. He explains of his dead friend, 'he can do magical things, like, you know, he can make it rain if... wants to, like, you know'. Whereas this narrative is generally rare within the white groups – maybe due to a Western narrative that does not give space to these kinds of notions – it was more common amongst ethnic minority users.

Spiritual accounts within the narratives seemed to have a more central role for Pakistani and Bangladeshi users. There was more of a connection made between their present circumstances and their faith and beliefs than for white users. Though psychiatry served an important role in their recovery, ultimately many felt at the mercy of God/Allah and only he could decide one's fate and future destiny. Whereas the younger Asian users were more concerned with being more 'disciplined' in reading the Koran and praying (which in itself gave them a sense of well-being), older Asian narratives emphasized the fight between good and evil – between good spirits and bad spirits. One user and her husband had been physically beaten by their in-laws who lived locally; she believed it was over inheritance, as the user had money and a house in Pakistan. She believed that her in-laws had made them mad through magic, this having been done by drinking water with a spell in it. As Yasmin explains,

> [The in-laws] said, 'drink the water after taking the prophet's name and stay inside and don't go out'. I didn't read the prayer or take the prophet's name but I drank it saying the name of Medina. Soon as I drank it I went mad. We (Yasmin and her husband) thought we were going to die anyway so if we were going to... die drinking the water of Medina, why not. So we drank it, both of us. We started fighting with each other. There was something strong in it, stronger than me. It said 'the declaration of faith' on top of the bottle but who knows what was in it. Our house went to pot. Everything was destroyed. For six months our house

> stayed empty. I was sent long distance to [the psychiatric hospital] and the police took our daughter. That's how cruel they were with us. That just happened recently, about two or three months ago. I've been going to [the psychiatric hospital] for 12 years. I stay a month or two months sometimes and still I don't get better. What can the doctors do?... If I give you a cold drink and it's got a spell in it how would you know? You wouldn't be able to find out. The doctors try and cure me but they can't understand why I don't get better. When I come home I'm back to stage one.

The spells are renewed when Yasmin's in-laws come,

> In my house and put spells in my house when I'm in hospital. My husband gave a key to his sisters. Look at this, all these things on the shelves, bottles, powders. Have you seen these dirty carrots? They're spells, that's what they've put there. They tell their brother what to do, 'do this', and he goes and does it.

The bad spells and spirits have been fought by prayer and by recital of parts of the Koran whilst asking for forgiveness for taking the 'bad water'. The bad magic tries to stop Yasmin and her husband from reading as well. She says of the magic, 'it felt like there was a stone on my chest which wouldn't let me go on the right path. Now it's as though I have permission to pray and read the Koran. There's blessing in those words'.

These narratives illustrate once more that periods of distress and crisis are very individual and given meaning in personalized ways. Psychiatry's paradox has been a failure to engage with these stories, hence the argument by some psychiatrists for a move towards narrative psychiatry as outlined in Chapter 2. Tariq's narrative (cited in Section 5.6) suggested the powers of a seer in that if he told people his dreams they would then come true. In some societies this is a revered status (see for instance Cohen 1988; Kleinman 1986, 1988). In the West there is more chance that you will be hospitalized and sedated. In Western psychiatry the power to define people as 'ill' and to treat them is firmly in the hands of the medical experts who 'know' and have the technical knowledge of these things. The user meanwhile preoccupies a lower status and is perceived as knowing very little about what they are experiencing, thus the user can only offer basic details which may facilitate the doctor's treatment decisions.

7.6 Positive aspects of illness

Despite a growing discourse suggesting positive aspects of mental health problems (including the 'artistic qualities' of manic depressives) only 11 of the 49 narratives mentioned anything that could fall under this heading. This included meeting good friends whilst being hospitalized, getting high on the medication and having a stronger sense of self. In the latter case, a number mentioned having more compassion for others and being more reflective about their own problems as a result of their crises. As Michael puts it,

> I think I've learned to relax a bit more about problems and see that everybody has problems, it's not just me with my problems. So I do feel a bit clearer in my thinking. Yeah, definitely more relaxed in my approach to problems and the way I want my life to be. The person I think I am, I feel I understand myself a lot better now.

There were a few users who felt they had experienced some 'beautiful things' and 'great feelings' whilst ill, as Philip comments, 'instead of having a headache, you'd have a bright sort of shiny feeling inside your head and that can come along anytime, and they [the conspirators] can give you that when they like'. However, the general feeling from the narratives was that this was not a good enough reason to stay 'ill'. Susie sums these feelings up:

> You do see things perhaps that other people can't see. But I would just rather be a normal person going to bingo with two-point-two kids and a fridge-freezer than this, you know. My doctor used to say to me, 'oh well, you're in good company – Van Gogh and Spike Milligan and Ludovic Kennedy'. And I'm not them. Do you know what I mean? I'm [Susie] in a council house. I'm a boring sod. As a single parent what am I doing? I'm not doing right good, you know.

7.7 The future

Most studies of mental health concentrate on the sufferings and sorrows of users, giving an inadequate picture of life beyond their illness. It is also important to highlight the forward-looking nature of many of the narratives rather than ignore these details. Parts of the narratives which touch on what users wanted to do next have been highlighted in Table 7.3.

Table 7.3 Future aspirations extracted from user narratives*

	Hospital	Home treatment	Total
Get a new job	8	2	10
Be well and avoid future crises	5	4	9
Move house/area	5	2	7
Go back to work	3	3	6
Study at college/university	4	1	5
Other	3	2	5
Do not know	3	2	5
Go on holiday	2	0	2

* Each user can appear in more than one category.

Future activities were cited in 32 of the user narratives. There was an obvious concern from some users to simply avoid 'relapse' or future periods of crisis. However, a priority for other users was to acquire some employment, whether voluntary, part-time or full-time. Indeed, some were waiting to re-enter their current jobs. There was also a wish amongst others to study further at college or university, both for self-fulfilment and for facilitating a more active social life and re-entry into the labour market. This is highlighted in a number of comments from users:

> First and foremost I'd like to be stabilized... with this and then I would like to go to college or something. There's all sorts of courses I fancy doing... In reality I'd like to... fill me time, you know I'd like to get back to work eventually. (Anita)

> I hope to work, you know, get a job and work. 'Cos... I mean there's no life without a job, which is true. (Jai)

> I'd rather be going back to work as soon as possible and getting back into a routine. That's what I'd rather do. I mean... but it's a vicious circle 'cos they, I don't know if it's the tablets that are makin' me sleepy... but they make me sleep, well, like, if you hadn't been coming today I wouldn't have gor up while 11:00.... But I think if you've got your work, your work takes up a lot o' time and then your leisure time, you fit it in better don't ya? You use it better... when I'm in routine of work... then I'm better able to do normal things. (Helen)

There were still problems in achieving these things but there were goals to aim for. Moving house or moving from the area – as well as going on holiday – were popular for a number of people, and appeared to be tied to an idea of a change of scenery and 'moving on' with one's life. In some cases, this was tied to where the user's extended family were based, such as Celia who talked of returning to where her mother lived in Surrey, which she believed would make 'a huge difference' to her life. A couple of users added their comments:

> Well, I just wish I could go on holiday somewhere. Then after the holidays... some kind of a job. You know, make my mind get a bit fresh and then... (Shakila)

> I'm hoping to move again some time. I don't particularly like this flat and it's got some bad memories for me, you know, actually living in here on me own and being ill. (Brian)

As has already been mentioned, there was some positivity among the BHTS users that things could happen for them in the future. Table 7.3 shows less future aspirations from these users, possibly suggesting that goals have already been achieved. Hospital-only users still have to deal with the difficulties which have been imposed by the medical psychiatric narrative. There were some who saw 'no future', as in the words of Zed, who had attempted to hang himself twice in the last month. But also some that felt the future held more promise than the immediate past, as Rachael commented, 'I've started dancing, yeah, I'm on the pull when I go out, looking for a new romance'.

7.8 Conclusion

Through performing a comprehensive content analysis of all the user narratives collected, a number of crucial issues have come to light. There are differentials between groups of users in terms of their own reflections on their lives which have been greatly influenced by psychiatry, from those believing they will always have periods of illness and are resigned to that fate through to those who see the illness as in the past and are concerned to look to the future. A fundamental finding has been that user self-definitions of their condition depend on the psychiatric care they receive. It was found that home treatment users are more likely to be able to redefine themselves into a 'less ill' or 'less severe' category and, thus, are able to redefine their illness biographies in a more positive way. At the same time, the crisis is not experienced as particularly positive for many of users. Further investigation of the self-definitions of illness showed development towards self-coping of crises by some, though the overbearing psychiatric narrative inhibits this for others. Spiritualism was also investigated and, particularly, for ethnic minority groups there is a suggestion that illness takes place externally to the body, meaning Western psychiatry is likely to be most inappropriate for these users. Finally, the user narratives cited a number of wishes for the future, with the majority expressing a desire to further reintegrate into society through entering the labour market, taking up education courses, socializing and getting out of the house more.

Along with Chapters 5 and 6, this chapter has raised some important new issues for mental health research and practice. In Chapter 8 the user narratives will be summarized, with recommendations being made for future ways of understanding and working with people experiencing mental health problems.

8
Conclusion

> So, all I want to do is, 'cos I get, I'll get like £85 a week and you're allowed, you're allowed to get that while you're over there, because it's common market. So I'll go to Greece, that'll pay for a room easily, like 50 quid a week to pay for a room. Plus then I'll like do some tweeky paintings for t'tourists, you know what I mean? Sit at side harbor and say, 'Oh, you can buy if you want, like'.
>
> (Alan)

8.1 Summary

This book had three main aims: to explore and demonstrate the possibility of taking a 'narrative approach' within medical and social research; to compare the narratives of users who obtained hospital-only treatment with users who received a new home treatment service; and to investigate periods of crisis (or 'illness') for those defined as acute or severe mental health users, with reference to their life stories (or 'narratives'). In this chapter the findings from the research will be summarized with reference to previous work and implications for the future will be drawn.

8.2 The 'narrative approach'

Mental health research has moved on from the early days of epidemiological studies to encompass more consumerist approaches. Surveys of user satisfaction are now commonplace, though they continue to surround the neo-liberalist agenda of meeting managerial targets rather than the humanitarian concern for investigation of patterns of care and illness. The social sciences have played an important role in critiquing medical practice in mental health, which has directly or indirectly supported groups of service users against the status quo (for example, Estroff 1981; Goffman 1961; Rosenhan 1996; Samson 1995a). The difference in the power relationship between social scientists and medical practitioners researching mental health users is a crucial factor in the evidence and insights that are gained. Whereas medical professionals have certain powers and privileges to maintain, the same is not true for social scientists, who are 'outsiders' looking in on medicine. The point is mentioned here because many of the studies of mental health user narratives/stories have come from inside the psychiatric profession. User life stories beyond this professional analysis have been left mainly to users themselves to publish independent accounts of mental health experience (for example, Coleman 1998; Read and Reynolds 1996), with Susko (1994: 87), suggesting that these accounts have had some effect on liberal psychiatrists developing 'narrative approaches' to treatment.

The 'narrative' definition chosen in this book followed Genette (1988) and Rosenau (1992) in relating it to peoples' 'stories' or 'life stories'. Whilst acknowledging the difficulties of extracting and reproducing the narrative as an accurate and 'true' account of the life experiences of users, the definition allowed a degree of flexibility in approaching personal constructions of reality. The 'methodology' chosen for the research was influenced by the work of Miller (1994), Denzin (1997) and Marcus (1994). Allowing the user to say anything they wanted was an attempt to move away from previous methodologies that tended to mould responses during interview, or to interpret and impose the writer's own narrative within analysis. Consequently, the texts reproduced varied enormously and it has been noted in Chapter 4 that some users adapted to this change in methodology better than others.

Personality theorists study narrative for explanations of actions and experience (see Section 2.6). Writers like Baumeister and Newman (1994) have stated that there are a limited number of reasons for a given narrative, such as seeking a notion of self-worth or justification and value for actions taken. However, the user narratives reproduced in this book have been much less concrete; the texts did not often state a particular reason for action or an understanding of an experience. In Section 5.6, for instance, Tariq outlined his violent behaviour towards his family, stating that he felt like someone else was controlling his body. Yet, later in the text, he denied that anyone would possess him with magic or spells. Tariq did not understand what happened to him or why he exhibited this behaviour. Such narratives cannot be seen simply as explanations for action. There is also a strong ideal within narrative approaches that inferences can be made towards generalizing patterns of human action and behaviour. This conflicts with the social constructionist and interpretative ethnographic influences in studying user narratives which call for the investigation of the *diversity* within the stories rather than seeking a *unified* narrative.

However, problems do arise with the narrative approach in relation to the continued presence of the researcher as the narrator of these life stories. It has been noted in Chapter 4 that a transcriber and a bilingual researcher were also involved in the transition from the immediacy of the user narrative to the analysis. Further translations of the resulting texts were then made by the author so as to present the results documented in Chapters 6 and 7. The content analysis in these chapters quantified the texts into tables and the narratives were, therefore, one stage further removed from the initial narrative witnessed by the researcher. So although we may claim to be 'acting as a scribe for the other', this does not mean that the final reproduced text is the actual narrative given. Agreeing with Frow and Morris (1993), the narrative is a 'lived text' not an account of actual 'lived experience'. What this lived text does is give a version of the narrative which is somewhat closer to the original view of the user than other methods allow.

In reaching the first aim of the book, it has been shown that the form of 'narrative method' applied in the research has been very useful in uncovering previously ignored personal constructions of life and, within this, the experiences of psychiatry. The method was produced through social constructionist and interpretative ethnographic discourse, as well as with reference to post-modernism, symbolic interactionism and Marcus's (1994) work on 'messy texts'. This has not brought about an 'abandonment of method', but rather further understanding of the researcher's relationship to the researched. Consequently, research that uses a narrative base will involve a significant amount of time in forward planning, collection of the narratives and, especially, analysis.

Given the current way social research is funded and carried out, it is debatable as to whether the resources will be available for many such narrative investigations in the future. If this is the case it will be to the detriment of future social research. Narrative study offers something quite different to other methods for it questions the researcher's own role in the exploration of social worlds. We are forced to question our own taken-for-granted assumptions that users of psychiatry – in this case – can only ever understand themselves in relation to their illness, or that a total focus on periods of user illness tells us all we need to know about the psychiatric system and mental health. Though evaluations can give efficient information about the benefits or otherwise of a new community service, the understanding of fundamental issues such as the nature of illness, health, coping or life trajectories (which can also help in long-term strategic planning) are lost to short-term outcomes.

8.3 Narrative comparisons

A second aim of this book was to compare home treatment user narratives with those people who experienced hospital care only. Although we attempted to match users like-for-like, the problems of the actual research process (see Chapter 4) meant more users – but less ethnic minorities – who had experienced hospital-only treatment were interviewed. Given the theoretical propositions behind the approach to narrative taken, each narrative is essentially different and it might seem that comparison would be a fruitless exercise. Comparison, however, did offer the opportunity to explore further the possibilities of the narrative approach and some of its limitations. For instance, without comparison we would not have found some essential differences in relation to life experiences and the effects that community psychiatric practices can have on user identities, such as the self-definitions of illness and the different perceptions of self-coping between the two groups.

Home treatment, the development of Crisis Resolution Teams and other forms of crisis intervention are seen from within as the 'evolution of psychiatry' from the asylum/psychiatric hospital with a medical model of care to the 'community' with its more 'humanistic' and 'holistic' approaches to treatment with users (see Clare 1982). It is recognized that replacing hospital wards with services in the community will not automatically mean a move to more socially orientated forms of care. Nevertheless, there is the assumption that a 'progression' in professional roles will take place as traditional models of care and treatment are challenged by the different environmental base in which professionals encounter users. The user narratives emphasized this environmental change. Instead of the user being presented to the professionals in the cold and sterile surroundings of the ward, the user received the professional(s) in his or her own home. The narrative form appeared to differentiate between the two groups of users, with home treatment narratives signalling that the treatment had to take account of their social problems due to the change in setting. The treatment options of medication and ECT offered in hospital contrasted with the socially orientated psychiatric narrative of home treatment. In the majority of cases this led to some consensus on treatment and the possibility of recovery.

What this narrative research has also shown is the ability of different psychiatric perspectives (or 'models of care') to alter user narratives in different ways. Broadly, the hospital-only user narratives repeatedly emphasized a biological base to their illness, medical treatment to suppress their symptoms and the real possibility of future periods of hospitalization at points of crisis (or 'relapse'). In contrast, home treatment user narratives suggested a more social base to crises, which meant the possibility of a fuller recovery and the ability to cope in the future without necessarily calling on psychiatric services. Like the hospital-only users, home treatment users were often on medication, yet in some cases these users were in search of 'alternative treatments' from counselling and psychotherapy to aromatherapy and spiritual healing. The Bradford Home Treatment Service users still had a fear of 'relapse', but outlined more ways in which crisis could be avoided. Succinctly put, it can be seen from these home treatment narratives that users were being proactive on the whole, whilst hospital-only users were mainly reacting to their periods of illness.

8.4 The psychiatric narrative and the user narratives

The research in this book has highlighted that what is perceived by medicine as accounts of 'psychiatric lives' is actually people's accounts of living and the effects of psychiatry on those lives. Other qualitative methodologies may have hinted at these themes, but quantitative accounts from users are much less likely to (Baumeister and Newman 1994). Although psychiatry has proved to be a dominant part of many users' lives, it is not the case for all. This was illustrated in Chapter 7 through differentiating between user texts which emphasized feelings of 'unwellness', 'getting by' or 'wellness'. Taking a narrative approach has produced some results that call for a fundamental reinterpretation of user experiences of psychiatric 'illness' and 'health'. The user narratives challenge the Western rational model of scientific medicine. The dominant biomedical approach within psychiatry works within a prescribed narrative of identification, diagnosis, treatment and cure of 'psychopathologies'. As we now summarize the results from Chapters 5, 6 and 7 with reference to these four major points of the dominant medical narrative, we will see that this positivistic narrative does not match with users' own understandings of their 'illnesses' or points of crisis.

8.4.1 Identification

From the 49 user narratives presented in this book it appears that identification of psychopathologies by psychiatry is no longer as important as it was during the epidemiological studies of the post-war years (Jodelet 1991; Scull 1984). Psychiatry's focus has changed from seeking to identify acute and severe forms of mental illness towards the identification of everyday pathologies (see Rose 1999). This includes the invention of new forms of everyday 'mental illness', often facilitated by the pharmaceutical multinationals (see Moynihan and Cassels 2005). The issues which dominate the acute sphere of mental health are the lack of acute beds and the management of this problem in each locale. Thus, referral routes to hospital or home treatment are vague and haphazard. Self or familial referral was common, as was referral from GPs, but – as one user noted – GPs may deal with user crises themselves without calling on any formal psychiatric intervention. In line with national trends (see Gomm 1996; Ramon 1996; Wilson 1999), ethnic minority users were more likely to be referred via police, and women via general hospital.

Given that nearly all of the users interviewed had received in-patient psychiatric treatment, it is unclear as to how psychiatrists made a distinction between those who were considered to be in 'acute' or 'severe' crisis and those who were not (that is, those who were considered by the consultants as needing home treatment or hospital care and those who were refused entrance on the grounds of suffering from a 'less severe' mental illness). Naturally, we remain unaware of the narratives of this latter population but consideration of diagnosis and behaviour of the users who were interviewed may enlighten this procedure of identification. Suffice to say that, given the shortage of acute beds, it is likely that such considerations are tempered by factors such as 'risk' to the community, support mechanisms available to the user in the home and other issues unrelated to the identification of particular 'psychopathologies' (see Pilgrim and Rogers 1996).

8.4.2 Diagnosis

When encountering a user for the first time, the medical classification manuals DSM IV (United States) and ICD 10 (rest of the world) allow the psychiatrist to identify the precise form of mental illness observed. This is what Susko (1994) calls the 'caseness approach'; groups of users are categorized under similar headings and this allows treatment to follow methodically on from formal diagnosis. A number of studies have shown the flaws in psychiatric attempts to accurately identify and diagnose psychopathologies (for example, Goffman 1961; Rosenhan 1996), which can lead to the labelling and stigmatization of everyday behaviour as evidence of abnormalities (Goffman 1963; Scheff 1996). It was illustrated in Chapter 7 that users have the ability to change their self-perceptions of their illnesses from 'psychotic' (for example, 'manic depression' or 'schizophrenia') to less severe forms of illness such as 'depression' or 'anxiety'. This result questions the possibility of fixed psychopathologies, or even whether such regimented psychopathologies exist at all (for example, Bracken and Thomas 1999b).

Following previous studies then, I would like to suggest that psychiatry is continuing to socially construct forms of psychopathology and justify these labels through a focus on the subjective reinterpretation of user behaviour. Thinking back to Rosenhan's (1996) study, his research students presented themselves to consultants complaining of hearing voices. All were subsequently admitted to psychiatric wards and given various psychotic labels. From the user narratives analysed in this research it is interesting that, again, hearing voices features prominently. Nearly all the narratives reproduced in Chapter 5, for example, mentioned hearing voices and, unsurprisingly, these users had previously been defined as 'psychotic' (usually 'schizophrenic'). It would appear that the hearing of voices is a clear sign to the psychiatrist of a systematic psychopathology, yet as was noted in Chapter 5 the narratives given vary considerably. For example, Rachael's voices were perceived as telling her to seek help for her (later diagnosed) cancer, yet this – together with her nightmares and hallucinations – was classified by the consultant as a part of her mental illness. Philip's voices were perceived as transmissions from his former work colleagues and the stealing of his thoughts. These voices were altogether more harmful for him, although he could also experience moments of chemical pleasure from the transmissions. His consultant, however, appeared more concerned about questioning Philip's relationship with his mother. It is particularly clear from a focus on the users who have experienced hospitalization that observed behaviour comes to be seen by medical staff as symptomatic of mental illness. Carmen's narrative expressed a battle with medical authorities throughout her life to avoid false diagnosis and treatment for her epilepsy. Her epileptic fits and behaviour, post-miscarriage, led to a diagnosis of 'hypermania'. Yunas and Tariq both experienced violent situations which led to physical and medical restraints as well as psychotic labels.

The consequences of such labelling behaviour can become a self-fulfilling prophecy – the downward spiral of being 'unwell', the possible loss of employment, family, friends and so on. People can become 'permanently sick' with a diminished social identity and a lack of social worth. The user narratives back the work of Barrett (1988) on consultants' writing behaviour, and Charon's (1992) and Showalter's (1992) work on the power of the consultant discourse, all of which reinforce the idea of a psychiatric narrative which dominates the personal narratives of users, redefining 'illness behaviour' into the language of medical science and psychopathology.

8.4.3 Treatment

Having identified and diagnosed behaviour as a form of mental illness, the logic of the biomedical model means a call for pharmacological treatment (with ECT being used where felt necessary) to control or eradicate symptoms. User behaviour is medicalized and redefined as a biochemical malfunctioning of the brain. Most of the users remained on medication, despite a number experiencing damaging side-effects. Some user narratives expressed positive outcomes from the medication: for Raiza the medication had dulled her voices; Tariq remarked that it had stopped him thinking about things; and Philip felt it was the only good thing he had got from his consultant. However, the home treatment user narratives suggest that such treatment options may have only a limited effect in dealing with peoples' circumstances. We have noted that many users felt there were fundamental social and economic reasons for their initial period of crisis, yet only medical options are utilized with hospitalized users. This is characterized by Philip's narrative (see Section 5.2), in which he suggests that what was really needed was for him to find a lawyer who believed him and would help him find the source of the conspiracy against him.

In support of Breggin (1993; see also in Miller 2006), we have also outlined user narratives in which medication can be a lethal straightjacket for users, disempowering them even to be able to speak about how they feel. Yunas's narrative (see Section 5.7) was quite profound on this point, believing that he 'woke up' once he was taken off his medication. He had had to read up himself on the dangers of taking the medication, which had not been explained to him by the medical staff. Yunas's experiences had left him concerned about 'relapse' and he had found it difficult to regain his sense of self. In a number of narratives – such as Gillian's (see Section 6.2) – the medication had caused the illness that was then seen as evidence of a pre-existing mental illness. The logic of the psychiatric narrative discounts real experience and pain as further evidence of the 'realness' of the user's 'psychopathology'. This might seem to confirm the thoughts of Derrida (1981) in that philosophies of science are incapable of reflecting on themselves in an original manner (though science believes it can reflect on the world in such a way). Psychiatry is part of the belief system of science which justifies its activities as 'scientific' through the myths of 'truth' and 'objectivity', and the use of a common unified narrative. Biomedical treatment can be deadly: there may be public outrage on the very rare occasions when a psychiatric user attacks a member of the public (see Muijen 1996), but users are regularly dying from the effects of years of medication (see Breggin 1993).

8.4.4 Cure

As was stated by Scull (1984) and others in Chapter 1, psychiatry has dispensed with the concept of 'curing' users before they leave hospital. However, the user narratives still expressed some ideal of being 'cured' or at least wanting to 'be well' again. Some users already perceived themselves as 'cured' (for example, Rachel's narrative in Section 5.4). This was mainly on the home treatment user side, and suggests the different professional narrative taken with users of the BHTS. It is also interesting to see that within the hospital-only user narratives, the language of the biomedical narrative ('relapse', 'controlling symptoms' and so on) has come to dominate the user's own narrative.

The psychiatric concept of 'cure' seems to have changed to the concept of 'control' (of symptoms, for example). Eradication of psychopathology no longer appears to be a goal for psychiatry, though the amount of research that continues to be carried out in bio-psychiatry – often with the cooperation and support of the pharmaceutical industries – suggests that they are still looking for the magic pill (for example, Breggin 1993). This may explain why some psychiatrists are willing to perceive themselves as being eclectic in their approaches to treatment (Samson 1995a) – so as to acknowledge some of the fallibilities of medical technologies.

A Western rational view of medicine follows the scientific aetiology of separating the mind from the body. However, it has been suggested by various writers on narratives that this may be to the detriment of understanding illness (for example, Peloquin 1993; Susko 1994). As if to confirm this, in Section 5.9, Raiza comments of 'feeling bad within myself':

> I was feeling that the left part of my body wasn't as good as the right part of my body is, you know... like good and bad. Things like that. It was all mixed up in my mind. I didn't know what I were doing.

Raiza's narrative appears to confirm the need to join the worlds of the mind and the body together to understand illness and the illness texts. If we at least start to take Kleinman's (1986, 1988) sociocentric view of illness seriously, we have more room in which to accept competing versions of reality rather than give precedent to one fixed model of reality which reduces mental problems to the malfunctioning of the brain. The narratives presented in this book do not, generally, back medical claims of the existence of 'mental illness'. The problem encountered in analysing such a variety of texts is further evidence of the dubious virtue of the psychiatric system. It could even be seen that the positive response to home treatment is due to the abandonment of the dominant psychiatric narrative and a move to a social narrative of user-orientated problem solving. However, even when we take out those users whose problems were more or less created by the psychiatric system and those who were mistakenly diagnosed with psychiatric disorders, there are still some people who are 'suffering'; we have witnessed narratives in which users have expressly talked of needing 'help' for their problems.

The user texts back a narrative approach as espoused by Gergen (1994) and Horner (1995) in Chapter 2. But one has to ask how this could work in Western society. The same theoretical research approach – adapted from social constructionism – in this book has not privileged any narrative, but could this be done in 'therapy sessions' by a group of professionals who have the power to dictate the treatment situation? Rose (1999) notes that Western society has become chained to the ideals of personal growth and personal responsibility: not only professionals but also the general public have accepted and internalized this psy-ideology. Could we really practise an approach which accepts competing versions of reality, truth and self-identity, when users have themselves internalized some fixed notions of 'being ill' and striving for 'normality'? If we worked with this interpretative view of the world then users would have to consider taking personal responsibility for their crises rather than believing the Western myth of 'professional help' within public arenas such as psychiatry. Although the user narratives may back the taking of such an approach, the logic of sociocentric views of the body cannot be followed through into practice. Foucault (1972) sees power as travelling in both directions. For instance, the psychiatrist has authority but this is also given to him or her by the users' own conceptions that this is the person that can help them. Is either side willing to give up this 'psy-pact'?

8.5 Ethnicity and gender

Ethnic minority groups remain over-represented in the mental health system (see MIND 2003; Wilson 1999). The reasons often given for this current state of affairs are Western psychiatry's inability to understand cultural differences and, more directly, the inherent racism of the psychiatric narrative (formed and maintained mainly by white middle-class males). Though we failed to obtain equal numbers of ethnic minority users in this research, these narratives were particularly negative towards psychiatry. Police intervention, a lack of support from professionals, bad experiences of hospital, high levels of medication and a lack of understanding towards the user all featured prominently.

These ethnic minority narratives were highlighted in Chapter 5, where the texts reproduced showed less 'personal understanding' outcomes than those of white users. This may suggest some cultural conflict, as confusion was particularly apparent within first-generation minority narratives. But our assessments of these narratives will inevitably be informed by our own Western understandings of illness and self, whereas this could be seen in completely different ways by the actual user. Spirituality was outlined in Chapter 7, and it appeared that particular beliefs could make more sense to some minority users than the medical model of disease. The influence of the psychiatric narrative on these personal meanings of illness may add to the internal confusion: we have witnessed narratives which have stated a position of 'not knowing' why certain behaviours have happened or what they might mean. That is, there is a possible contradiction between the idea that the user is 'ill' and has a 'disease' of the mind, compared to a personal understanding that may, for example, emphasize the possession of bad spirits within the body. A conflict between personal and professional illness narratives arise, as well as a conflict between Eastern and Western cultural narratives of understanding.

Younger minority users – usually second generation – may also experience a cultural confusion, having internalized two sets of competing values (Eastern and Western). This could materialize as generational conflict, as Raiza's narrative (see Section 5.9) expressed a concern that she was not 'fitting in' with other people. It could also be understood as a part of the difficulty in living by a set of values handed down from older generations, whilst being assimilated in the values of Western society. As second-generation British Asian writer and performer Meera Syal has commented, 'for us every step is a new one. It's different for the people below us and it's different for our parents. We are the generation that is sort of creating the new culture' (Grindrod 1999: 19). More obviously, young Black and Asian people are experiencing difficulties in obtaining opportunities in education and employment, and are more prone to being socially excluded from mainstream culture (for example, Green *et al.* 2001).

Hospitalization appears even less appropriate for ethnic minority users than for white users, and from the narratives witnessed the institution would seem to serve as little more than a holding house for them. Home treatment narratives from minority users expressed some positivity about the avoidance of the hospital and also the prevalence of minority staff on the team who might better understand them. For example, recognition was made by the BHTS staff members of daily prayers and readings of the Koran, which could become one form of self-help for practising Muslim users.

Like ethnic minorities, women tend to be over-represented in the psychiatric system (Gomm 1996). Reference can again be made to the fact that those with the power to refer and treat users within the medical profession are usually male. Roughly equal numbers of males and females were present in the current research, and from the female narratives there is evidence that experience and behaviour continues to be medicalized within psychiatry. A number of female narratives, for example, emphasize some loss (of relationships, babies or even the will to live), yet diagnosis and treatment emphasized an illness of the mind. There was a misinterpretation of events by psychiatry, with personal problems and physical illnesses being seen as evidence of 'mental illness' as well as a tendency to reclassify women's behaviour as 'mad' rather than 'bad' (see for instance Carlen 1988). Often the experience is gendered, so that women with anorexia, epilepsy, breast cancer and so on can find themselves on a psychiatric ward and on high dosages of medication.

8.6 Social and economic factors

It has been argued that poverty and social deprivation are key variables in the descent into mental illness, the question is whether this is middle-class stereotyping of the working classes or whether the illness is the consequence of the stress experienced (for example, Pill and Stott 1986). Generally, the narratives invoked additional antagonisms for working-class people: for men, these were seen in the context of a macho working-class culture which involved heavy drinking, violence and manual labour. For working-class women it could be a narrative which involved looking after a family and experiencing difficult – sometimes emotionally or physically violent – relationships. A difference in social and economic backgrounds between hospital and BHTS users has been noted elsewhere (see Cohen 1999a). As an indicator, when interviewing home treatment users the researchers were more likely to be travelling to 'better areas' of the city and, occasionally, into the suburbs. This may signify more of a likelihood of working-class people ending up in hospital with acute or severe illness labels and the further pathologizing of working-class values and behaviour by middle-class professionals (for more on class and cultural conflict, see for example, Miller 1958).

A theme that has run through this book, echoed by the user narratives themselves, is the significance of social and economic life factors for the users of psychiatry. Internal and external critiques of the biomedical approach have pointed to the inability of psychiatry to look at the factors that surround people when crises are presented to them. The research in this book backs up previous studies (for example, Kleinman and Good 1985; Mitchell 1969; Pill and Stott 1986), with constant references made to the influence of social factors in leading to a crisis, as well as possibly offering a way out of the crisis. Despite this, psychiatry's ability to adapt to these findings remains muted. The user narratives highlighted many precipitating factors including family and relationship problems, financial, education and work issues, and also problems with drink or drugs. The significance of these factors was again highlighted in Section 7.6, when activities for the future were mentioned. These included obtaining employment or restarting work, moving house and taking up studies at college or university. Significantly, home treatment users mentioned fewer issues for the future than hospital users. This may well be because home treatment psychiatry had actually spent time addressing some of these issues with the users as part of their 'social' form of care.

The hospital does offer some temporary social and economic comfort in terms of the possibility of meeting friends on the ward and not having to pay for heating, meals and so on, for the duration of the user's stay. Like all psychiatric hospitals, there was also an Approved Social Worker on site who helped users sort out financial and familial matters, yet the author failed to find one reference to such a person in the narratives. As we have seen, hospital generally offers limited solutions to users' long-term problems, which may have precipitated hospitalization and will possibly have to be faced on return to the 'community'. Given the limited engagement with ward staff and the lack of concern showed by some of them, it is not so surprising that hospital-only narratives expressed a degree of pessimism about the future.

Not only is the success of home treatment psychiatry significant in exposing the ineffectuality of biomedical psychiatry to help users, but also the evidence from the user narratives expressed a wide range of self-coping mechanisms that were related to their everyday lives and not necessarily to pharmaceutical products. The self-coping mechanisms cited usually overlapped: work, for instance, also became a part of being able to socialize and interact with others as well as gain confidence and more self-esteem. Going out – remembering the a number of users felt agoraphobic – could also help build a user's confidence: shopping (leisure or essential), walking in the park and visiting others were seen as therapeutic and, in some cases, this increased the user's feelings of independence. In a number of forms, the arts allowed expression of personal feelings and a degree of relaxation. Even simple things like 'stroking the dog' was preferable to another dose of psychiatry (see Section 7.3). As has been mentioned before, these coping mechanisms are the taken-for-granted parts of our lives. They could almost be seen as 'naturally occurring' events in most peoples' lives – through constantly created and recreated images of how we should live, these events have become omnipresent (Rose 1999; Turner 1995). Yet, the logic of the biomedical model fails to engage with these 'therapies'. It may be because these are activities that lay people can perform which do not involve professional intervention or it might be because these self-interventions are seen as secondary to medical causes and solutions for illness.

Narratives from the BHTS users have shown that understanding the user's social and economic issues can facilitate some recovery from the crisis (even if there is still some emphasis on pharmacological treatment). It is to the detriment of psychiatry that social and economic life factors continue to be marginalized or ignored. We now have examples of user narratives where improvements in psychiatry's way of working (in this case, through the BHTS) can achieve some success.

8.7 Metaphor and meaning

Another interesting finding from the user narratives was the way in which certain metaphors were used to represent being 'ill' or 'healthy'. For instance, Michael's narrative (see Section 5.3) was a search for the 'light at the end of the tunnel'. Depression for Michael was a 'downward spiral'; he believed that 'things are that deep' that he would need a few years of counselling to sort out his problems. Further, he stated that he had been going 'round and round in circles' previously with his depression, but he could now see 'a bit of straight road'. Illness, therefore, can also be represented as a deep descent of the self, whilst being healthy (or 'normal' as some users put it) was represented by the main road to which one must return. The 'deep' metaphor was often mentioned by users in their narratives, as was the 'spiralling' and 'being out of control' metaphors. Metaphors of this nature can be used within psychiatry as they are in other professions (for examples from magistrates and the police, see Brown 1991a, 1991b; Cohen 1996). This suggests further evidence of the domination of the professional narrative over the personal narrative. It can also be seen, however, as an attempt by users to visualize and create meaning for what has come to be considered a period of 'illness' (see Herzlich and Pierret 1986). If a user narrative talks in metaphors such as 'spiralling out of control', for instance, it also facilitates a self-reflection of a flow along an imagined illness–health trajectory. Thus, if one feels aware of 'falling down', one can in the same way pick oneself 'back up' again. This is just a couple of possible views on the content of the illness metaphors and, obviously, they may mean something quite different to the user. This view does, however, fit well with Gergen's (1994) emphasis within the narratives on personally constructed periods of 'highs' and 'lows'.

8.8 Implications

A number of users had no complaints whatsoever with their treatment and nothing but praise for their experiences of the local mental health services in Bradford. Of course we know psychiatry has had a chequered history and that some problems remain, but one cannot deny that people want and need psychiatric help from time to time. This argument, like many of those centred on incarcerated communities, appears to be approaching socially defined problems and differences the wrong way around. It is the very history of psychiatry that is important to its current position, with the mental health professionals acquiring the cultural, medical and scientific capital to be seen as the 'experts' in the field. For if someone is seen to be acting 'oddly', we know we can take that person to the 'experts' rather than that person having to cope on their own. This is akin to Weber's (1958) 'iron cage' of a tightening bureaucracy in a society of self-regulation, where professional intervention is preferred to laissez-faire (see Rose 1999; Samson 1995b). We have seen from this research that psychiatry has a myth of choice – the choice of treatment, to engage with staff, to accept diagnosis, to change doctors and so forth – whereas in reality there is little choice. The bottom line remains biomedical treatment. This brings us back to Samson's (1995a) 'medico-eclecticism' within psychiatry – the appearance of pragmatic eclecticism in treating mental health problems but an underlying faith in the biomedical model, justified by the appearance of a 'reformed' approach to mental health care.

Further, there is evidence that user narratives of illness and coping are interrupted by the dominant psychiatric narrative (or a modernized version through home treatment). Within the psy-complex there still remain countless ways of interpreting and categorizing behaviour, and the arguments continue as to the specific symptoms which inform each category of psychiatric 'disorder' (for example, Samson 1995b). The underlying knowledge base that marks out this group of professionals has yet to be made clear, yet psychiatry is allowed to continue. Hopefully, the research in this book has made it clear that there are as many different people as problems, that psychiatric labelling of mental health users stigmatizes rather than facilitates recovery, that the understanding of the self is very personal, and that we can only gain some hermeneutic insights into what these patterns of internal understanding might be – 'traces of local knowledge' as Geertz (1983) has put it.

Explanations for behaviour described as 'mental illness' may take us in many different directions. This is where Foucault's analysis is tremendously useful, centring as it does on the use of language by different groups. Whilst language is utilized by psychiatry to create the illusion of medical realities such as 'schizophrenia' or 'post-traumatic stress disorder', users are both guided by this narrative and, simultaneously, interpreting their experience in ways which occasionally resist these realities. User narratives both reflect the wider dimensions of power and the individual attempts to reconstruct a self. Herzlich and Pierret (1986: 91) add that in most societies, conceptions of illness oscillate between the attack of external factors to the self and the illness being seen as 'within the individual'. The mental health user narratives that have been investigated suggest that there is a constant interplay between mind and body – external and internal constructions – in the creation of the 'illness' experience.

Projects such as the BHTS held a special place within local psychiatric services for a few years, but has subsequently been altered to fit with the UK government's latest policies for the development of Crisis Resolution Teams. The Bradford Crisis Resolution Home Treatment Team continues to offer 24-hour, 7-days-a-week intensive input at home, but its defining principles of being a needs-led alterative to hospitalization have been partially lost. The BHTS was a success; it introduced a different model of care and the staff succeeded in reducing medication levels in a sizeable proportion of cases, as well as discouraging the use of ECT (see Bracken and Cohen 1999; Cohen 1999a). Yet the 'post-psychiatric' project had many opponents, both locally and nationally. It was once commented to me by a consultant that you cannot have 'socialism in one country'. In other words, the whole system has to change otherwise the one 'socialist state' (in this case the BHTS) that uses a different model of care will be swept aside by opposing forces (meaning, the psychiatric hospital, the CMHRCs, the social services, the Health Trust management and other parts of the local mental health care system). This appears to have been the case.

Nevertheless, the reproduced texts have shown that, if users are given the space to talk and be heard by mental health workers, this can create a more equal situation in which to understand problems of living. In the case of the BHTS, this process was also facilitated by the change in location from hospital to the home, which witnessed the exchange of some power back to the user and the user's family. In Chapter 5, however, it was noted that a 'joint narrative' was not always agreed upon, and sometimes the user narrative was again in conflict with a psychiatric narrative. Catriona's narrative (see Section 5.5), for example, outlined what she perceived as unnecessary interference from home treatment psychiatry. This suggests that the 'narrative approach' in psychiatry is conditional on acceptance of certain attributes and behaviour that is seen as 'for the best' or 'in the user's best interests'. Non-cooperation, therefore, can lead to the more hard-line biomedical model and hospitalization. Catriona's narrative centred on her anger and frustration at the whole system of psychiatry, and home treatment in this case was seen as just another part of that system.

This evidence of conflict between the user and the health worker suggests there are limits not only to the 'social approach' but, more specifically, the 'narrative approach' within psychiatry. There is a continued imbalance within treatment which is likely to continue as long as the professionals with the power to prescribe medication, to hospitalize and to section users are the same ones directly responsible for the 'care' of users (in this respect, it is positive to see the UK government currently tackling the power of consultants in the RMO role, see Department of Health 2007). The BHTS claimed to be 'user-orientated' or 'user-centred' within their approach, yet a conflict remained in terms of the differentials of power and control involved in the process of care. The user is given more authority and say in their process of recovery only if they agree to engage with the professional narrative which informs the home treatment approach (such as having socially orientated solutions, but also drawing on medication where felt necessary; negotiating issues of 'risk'; and consideration of family and carer roles). If a user fails to 'engage' on this basis, the role of the user may be diminished.

Without the centrality of the user in the process of 'treatment', there is less chance of the user avoiding a subsequent period of psychiatry in the future. Therefore, the more individualized the care received and the less the 'caseness' approach is taken, the more likely it is that positive long-term outcomes can be achieved. We have witnessed hospital-only user narratives which sometimes mirrored Goffman's (1961) 'moral careers' of sustained periods of hospitalization – sometimes stretching over a lifetime – but we have also seen that those with the BHTS could assert more positive ways of living in the future without psychiatric support.

8.9 Conclusion

Mental health professionals only achieve their status through a narrative of 'expertise' in being the appropriate people to treat the problems of both mind (usually interpreted as the brain) and body. If reflexivity was possible within the profession it would be acknowledged that psychiatry has achieved surprisingly little in terms of positive, long-term outcomes for users. Professionals who work with user-centred approaches and a narrative method can at least begin to understand individual problems, but there also needs to be a limited period of interaction with the user, assisting them to attain a 'life of wellness' (a social life, employment, points of relaxation and so on). We live in a world involving a close 'governing of the self' (Rose 1999), we are all affected by the search for understanding and meaning to our periods of distress. Though medical science may have created the facades of 'illness' and 'health', it has become a personal reality for us. Users need to be encouraged to develop the use of day-to-day activities as resources to self-cope with trauma, rather than draw repeatedly on psychiatric professions and medical treatment which can come to dominate their own ability to cope and live independently. The dominant psychiatric narrative exists and traumatizes, but within it there are possibilities for resistance in which burgeoning crisis intervention projects like the ill-fated BHTS can address local issues of user problems in living.

The research in this book has demonstrated that – with the aid of both new and old theoretical approaches from the social sciences – studying disadvantaged and marginalized people through a 'narrative approach' can highlight new and burgeoning issues that place both the researcher and those studied within a joint research text. It has also been shown that what is defined as 'mental illness' can be experienced in many different ways, depending on such factors as meaning, experience, agency, social and economic life worlds, and conceptions of self. These new approaches to illness and recovery as defined by the users themselves need to be taken seriously by health care professionals in their day-to-day work. What is also clear is that a period of distress or crisis which has led to psychiatric intervention can both empower and disadvantage users depending on the different models of psychiatric care received.

Further, the research has shown that the user narratives can change according to the form of psychiatric narrative entailed in the treatment, leading to some change of personal identity from an ideal of 'being well' to an identity of 'being unwell'. Until there is a perceived alternative to the psychiatric narrative (and with it the power and dominance of the biomedical model) there will be a continual submergence of the individual illness narrative. In a plea for reform, Kleinman (1988: 266–7) has commented,

> If we can say that war is too important to be left solely to generals and politics solely to politicians, then we should also say that illness and care are far too important to be left solely in the hands of medical professionals, especially those who configure those innate human issues in a framework that constrains our humanity.

Finally, it is relevant to add that there is a need for more research which surveys the broader context of a person's life world in attempting to understand perceived notions of illness. Medical and social researchers should be encouraged to experiment further with forms of narrative study to produce a new range of analytical devices which can aid our understanding of people and society. Just as importantly, it is relevant to take this research forward into the public and professional arenas both in and outside of medicine and sociology to offer alternative accounts of mental health to those that predominate in our society and, thus, to promote further understanding of this very individual form of distress.

Appendices

A.1 Initial letter given to all Bradford Home Treatment Service users at discharge

[Date]

Dear [name]

We have employed a researcher to look at the care you have received from the Bradford Home Treatment Service and also your general experiences of psychiatry. He will be interviewing a number of people and it is possible that he will contact you soon. If so, we hope that you will be willing to be interviewed.

If you are selected for interview, you will be sent a letter by the researcher to ask if you are willing to take part. If you have any questions you can contact him, Bruce Cohen, at the University of Bradford on 01274-384781.
Best wishes,

Yours sincerely

Dr Pat Bracken Dr Phil Thomas

A.2 Letter sent to sampled home treatment users, requesting an interview

[Name]
[Address]

[Date]

Dear [name]

As you may know the Bradford Home Treatment Service is still very much in its infancy and the Bradford Community Health NHS Trust, through the University of Bradford, have employed me to carry out an independent evaluation of the Bradford Home Treatment Service. I am particularly concerned to get *your views* on what you thought of the home treatment service, your comments will help to develop the service in the future so that it can better meet the needs of fellow users. To this end, I would be very grateful if you would agree to an interview/discussion with me about the Bradford Home Treatment Service. The interview should take no longer than 30–45 minutes and will be anonymous – nobody other than the research team will know who said what in each interview.

I would like to draw your attention to the enclosed information sheet which the Trust has asked me to include with this letter, which gives some more explanation about the reason for these interviews.

If you have a telephone, I will be calling you in the next few days with the possibility of arranging an interview at your home in the near future. If you have no telephone and would like to be interviewed, please fill in the details below, including giving any times when you are available for an interview and I will send you details of when I will call (alternatively you can phone me on 01274-384781). I hope you will see the value of taking part in this study and thank you in advance for your time.

Yours sincerely,

Bruce M Z Cohen (Research Assistant)

Only fill this part in if you have no telephone and would like to be interviewed:

Name ....

Days/Times I am available...

Any special requirements? (e.g. translator, etc.).................................

PLEASE RETURN TO:

BRUCE M Z COHEN

DEPARTMENT OF SOCIAL & ECONOMIC STUDIES

UNIVERSITY OF BRADFORD BD7 1DP

PATIENT INFORMATION SHEET

The Bradford Community Health NHS Trust has established a new service in the south west sector of the city. This is the area served by the Ashgrove Resource Centre. It is important with new developments like this that patients and carers' views of the service are fully taken into account. With this in mind a research project has developed to monitor the new service.

As well as interviewing patients who have been treated by the new service we are also anxious to compare the new service with more traditional hospital treatment. With this in mind a number of people who have recently been in-patients in [hospital] will be asked to participate in this study.

Each interview will take approximately one hour and will be tape recorded. You will not be asked to fill in any forms or questionnaires. You will be asked about your views on the care received and your satisfaction with this care. If you have a carer you will be asked about the care received by your relative/friend and the support given by the services to yourself.

While your help with this monitoring project would be most appreciated, if you do not feel able to participate this will in no way affect the care you receive from either the Home Treatment Service or the hospital. You are completely free to refuse to be interviewed.

If you agree to be interviewed the researcher will contact you to arrange a suitable time and place for the interview to take place.

The tape-recorded interviews will remain confidential and will only be listened to by the researcher and his supervisors. Interviews will be transcribed but the patient or carers name will not be entered. Thus it will not be possible to identify the subject of the interview in any report.

A.3 Letter sent to hospital-only users requesting an interview

[Name]
[Address]

[Date]

Dear [name]

I have been employed by the Bradford Community Health NHS Trust to do an independent evaluation of the general experiences of ex-psychiatric patients in the area. I am writing to ask if you would be able to take part in an interview with myself. As a former patient of [the psychiatric hospital] your experiences are particularly important in helping us assess the effectiveness of such provision in Bradford.

The interviews are carried out at your convenience. If you have any special requirements (such as a bilingual or female researcher), we would be happy to accommodate these. The interviews are confidential and anonymous. No names are given when reporting back from interviews. Taking part in the interview will in *no way* effect your possible future use of psychiatric or other health services, and you are free to withdraw from the interview at any time.

Could you kindly fill in your response and send back the bottom part of this letter in the enclosed reply-paid envelope. Alternatively, if you are on the telephone, I will be in touch shortly. If there are any further queries you have regarding the research, please feel free to phone me, Bruce Cohen, at the University of Bradford on 01274-384781.

Yours sincerely

Bruce M Z Cohen, Mental Health Researcher

I ***do/do not*** *wish to take part in an interview [please delete as appropriate]*
I would prefer to be interviewed on ....[date] at .... [time].
I would prefer a bilingual researcher □ *[please tick if applicable]*
Please state your preferred language if ***not*** *English:.............................*
Contact telephone number: ....

A.4 Background information, notes and draft topic guide for pilot interviews

Aims of questionnaire with users

- To elicit the personal meanings and interpretations of the periods of 'psychiatric illness' that users give to their experience (explanations or conceptions of illness).
- To discover whether home treatment users give value/difference to particular home treatment experiences. And whether this has altered their general view of coping, well-being and of psychiatry.

- To elicit an assessment of treatment on both home treatment and psychiatric hospital, both positive and negative. To be able to reflect on hospital experience (if they have one).
- To discover a person's life history as it is individually perceived, and investigate periods of crisis in a person's life, including the strategies they use to be able to cope during such periods (whether self, social or professional coping strategies) and to look at the factors facilitating recovery.
- To elicit accounts of the effects that (1) the illness and (2) psychiatric treatments of illness has had on user lives.
- To investigate current user feelings about their lives, and health/illness in the future.

Themes for user questionnaire

- Psychiatric experience.
- Periods of coping and non-coping.
- Periods of health and illness.
- Life experience (points of crisis within it) – the life story.
- Likes, dislikes, traits – how would they describe themselves?
- Being in the world – how they see themselves.
- Safety/non-safe environments – feelings of safety.
- Social support/family support.
- Self-disclosure and research process – why they tell me, what they *feel* about disclosing stuff to me.
- Current/future hopes and fears – assessment of their current mental health.
- Life changes (education, work, personal).
- Help-seeking.
- Self-explanation of illness – What was it like? What did it feel like to them?
- Self-definition of 'illness' – label.
- How were they perceived by psychiatry?
- How they perceive themselves in relation to the rest of society.

Notes for topic guide design

Gergen and Gergen: Looked at points of crisis for people (highs and lows).

Estroff: Uses questionnaire... areas of study may be useful – unemployment, employment, general living circumstances, social life, friends, people at work, neighbours, housework, work history, parents/family, religion, community, finances, shopping, transport, housing, professionals.

Kleinman: Meanings relate to a worsening crisis... at certain critical points in the life course.

Miller: Did 90-minute open-interview, using a minimal structure/prodding, users simply asked to talk about themselves.

NB: User needs to have right to pull out of interview at any time, socio-demographic stuff can get from the monitoring forms – don't want to raise these factors as issues during interviews unless user raises them.

Contents to put in topic guide

- Life experiences – periods of highs and lows (crises) within it.
- How they coped with points of crisis? (self, social, professional).
- Brief psychiatric history (as they see it) – hospital/home treatment experience – was value gained from being in hospital/on home treatment? What are their feelings towards the benefits of psychiatry, or the drawbacks of psychiatry?
- Effects of illness on their lives.
- How they feel about themselves and their experiences now.
- Their current attitude to their lives – positive? negative? ambivalent?
- How they see their future.
- How they might cope with future crisis (has psychiatry been of long-term benefit to them?).

Topic guide

(1) I am very interested in finding out more about your life history as you perceive it. What do you see as the crucial points in your life (education, work, personal life, etc.)?
(2) When there were crisis points in your life, how did you deal/cope with them (self, social, professional help)?
(3) Could you tell me about your experiences of psychiatry? What were the periods in hospital like? (if applicable) What were your periods on home treatment like (environment, staff, treatment, etc.)?
(4) Do you feel there is anything you have gained from your experiences of psychiatry (dealing with crises/illness, etc.)?
(5) How do you feel generally about yourself and your life at present (work, unemployment, personal life, relations with others)?
(6) Do you have any plans for the future (health, work, education, social, etc.)?
(7) If you have any future crises in your life, how do you see yourself coping/dealing with them (psychiatry – any effect on this)?

A.5 Revised topic guide following pilot interviews

(1) Do you remember the first time you used a psychiatric service? How did this come about?
(2) What did you feel that you needed from psychiatry (medication, support, etc.)?
(3) Generally, how have you found the experience of using psychiatry? Have they been positive?
(4) (If applicable) How would you compare your experiences of home treatment with your experiences of hospital (similarities? differences?)?
(5) Do you feel there is anything you have gained from your experiences of psychiatry (dealing with crises/illness, etc.)?
(6) How do you feel generally about yourself and your life at present (work, unemployment, personal life, relations with others)?
(7) What would you like to do in the future (health, work, education, social, etc.)?
(8) If you have any future crises in your life, how do you see yourself coping/dealing with them (psychiatry – any affect on this?)?

Bibliography

Abbott, A. (1993) 'Measure for measure: Abell's narrative methods', *Journal of Mathematical Sociology*, 18, 2–3, 203–14.

Abell, P. (1984) 'Comparative narratives: some rules for the study of social action', *Journal for the Theory of Social Behaviour*, 14, 3, 309–31.

Abell, P. (1987) *The Syntax of Social Life*, Oxford: Oxford University Press.

Abell, P. (1993) 'Some aspects of narrative method', *Journal of Mathematical Sociology*, 18, 2–3, 93–134.

American Psychiatric Association (2003) APA Statement on "Diagnosis and Treatment of Mental Disorders", Press Release No. 03–39, 26 September, http://www.mindfreedom.org/know/mental-health-activism/2003/mf-hunger-strike/hunger-strike-debate/apa-2nd-reply-to-mfi (accessed 2 March 2007).

Anderson, A. and Goolishian, H. (1992) 'The client is the expert: a not-knowing approach to therapy', in McNamee, S. and Goolishian, H. (eds) *Therapy as a Social Construction*, Newbury Park: Sage.

Armstrong, D. (1983) *Political Anatomy of the Body: Medical Knowledge in Britain in the Twentieth Century*, Cambridge: Cambridge University Press.

Audini, B., Marks, I. M., Lawrence, R. E., Connolly, J. and Watts, V. (1994) 'Home-based versus out-patient/in-patient care for people with serious mental illness: Phase II of a controlled study', *British Journal of Psychiatry*, 165, 204–10.

Audit Commission (1994) *Finding a Place: A Review of Mental Health Services for Adults*, London: HMSO.

Bachelard, G. (1984) *The New Scientific Spirit*, Boston: Beacon Press.

Bailey, S. (1994) 'Bradford crisis services: where are they?', *Open Mind*, 72, 15.

Banton, R., Clifford, P., Frosh, S., Lousada, J. and Rosenthall, J. (1985) *The Politics of Mental Health*, London: Macmillan.

Barbre, J. W. and Personal Narratives Group (1989) 'Origins', in Barbre, J. W. and Personal Narratives Group (eds) *Interpreting Women's Lives*, Bloomington and Indianapolis: Indiana University Press.

Barham, P. and Hayward, R. (1991) *Relocating Madness: From the Mental Patient to the Person*, London: Tavistock/Routledge.

Barron, P. (2001) '"Postpsychiatry" is Psychiatry in Learning Disabilities', *British Medical Journal* (online), 24 March, http://www.bmj.com/cgi/eletters/322/7288/724#13443 (accessed 1 March 2007).

Barrett, R. J. (1988) 'Clinical writing and the documentary construction of schizophrenia', *Culture, Medicine and Psychiatry*, 12, 265–99.

Baumeister, R. F. and Newman, L. S. (1994) 'How stories make sense of personal experience: motives that shape autobiographical narratives', *Personality and Social Psychology Bulletin*, 20, 6, 676–90.

BBC (2002) 'All in the mind: Bradford', 16 October, http://www.bbc.co.uk/radio4/science/allinthemind_20021016.shtml (accessed 19 February 2007).

BBC (2005) 'Voices', http://www.bbc.co.uk/northyorkshire/voices2005/glossary/glossary.shtml (accessed 19 March 2007).

BBC (2007) 'Secrets of the drug trials', 29 January, http://news.bbc.co.uk/2/hi/programmes/panorama/6291773.stm (accessed 5 March 2007).

Bean, P. and Mounser, P. (1993) *Discharged From Mental Hospitals*, London: Macmillan.

Bengelsdorf, H., Church, J. O., Kaye, R. A., Orlowski, B. and Alden, D. C. (1993) 'The cost effectiveness of crisis intervention: Admission diversion savings can offset the high cost of service', *The Journal of Nervous and Mental Disease*, 181, 12, 757–62.

Beumont, P. J. V. (1992) 'Phenomenology and the history of psychiatry', *Australian and New Zealand Journal of Psychiatry*, 26, 532–45.

Botting, F. (1995) 'Culture, subjectivity and the real; or, psychoanalysis reading postmodernity', in Adams, B. and Allan, S. (eds) *Theorizing Culture*, London: UCL Press.

Bracken, P. (2001) 'The radical possibilities of home treatment: postpsychiatry in action', in Brimblecombe, N. (ed.) (2001) *Acute Mental Health Care in the Community: Intensive Home Treatment*, London: Whurr.

Bracken, P. (2002) 'Depression, psychiatry and the use of ECT', *Asylum* (online), 12, 4, http://www.asylumonline.net/archive/v12_n4_26-28.htm (accessed 19 February 2007).

Bracken, P. and Cohen, B. M. Z. (1999) 'Home treatment in Bradford', *Psychiatric Bulletin*, 23, 6, 349–52.

Bracken, P. and Thomas, P. (1998) 'A new debate in mental health', *Open Mind*, 89, 17.

Bracken, P. and Thomas, P. (1999a) 'Home treatment in Bradford, *Open Mind*, 95, 17.

Bracken, P. and Thomas, P. (1999b) 'Let's scrap schizophrenia', *Open Mind* (online) 99, reproduced at http://www.critpsynet.freeuk.com/Sept99.htm (accessed 2 March 2007).

Bracken, P. and Thomas, P. (1999c) 'Post-psychiatry: science, psychiatry and the mystery of madness', *Open Mind*, 100, 10–11.

Bracken, P. and Thomas, P. (2001) 'Postpsychiatry: a new direction for mental health', British Medical Journal (online), 322, 724–7, http://www.bmj.com/cgi/content/full/322/7288/724 (accessed 2 March 2007).

Bradford Home Treatment Service (1996) *Operational Policy*, Bradford: Bradford Community Health NHS Trust.

Breggin, P. (1993) *Toxic Psychiatry*, London: Harper Collins.

Brimblecombe, N. (2001) 'Community care and the development of intensive home treatment services', in Brimblecombe, N. (ed.) *Acute Mental Health Care in the Community: Intensive Home Treatment*, London: Whurr.

Brown, S. (1991a) *Magistrates at Work: Sentencing and Social Structure*, Buckingham: Open University Press.

Brown, S. (1991b) *On the Brink of the Slippery Slope: Magistrates' Discourse, Sentencing and Youth Control*, Paper presented at the British Criminology Conference 1991, Middlesbrough: Teesside Polytechnic.

Bruner, J. (1986) *Actual Minds, Possible Worlds*, Cambridge: Harvard University Press.

Burti, L. and Tansella, M. (1995) 'Acute home-based care and community psychiatry', in Phelan, M., Strathdee, G. and Thornicroft, G. (eds) *Emergency Mental Health Services in the Community*, Cambridge: Cambridge University Press.

Bynum, W. F. (1981) 'Rationales for therapy in British psychiatry, 1780–1835', in Scull, A. (ed.) *Madhouses, Mad-Doctors and Madmen: The Social History of Psychiatry in the Victorian Era*, London: The Athlone Press.

Cabrera-Abreu and Milev (2001) 'The sleep of reason produces monsters', *British Medical Journal* (online), 26 March, http://www.bmj.com/cgi/eletters/322/7288/724#13490 (accessed 1 March 2007).

Canguilhem, G. (1994) 'The death of man, or exhaustion of the cogito?', in Gutting, G. (ed.) *The Cambridge Companion to Foucault*, Cambridge: Cambridge University Press.

Caplan, G. (1964) *Principles of Preventative Psychiatry*, New York: Basic Books.

Capra, F. (1982) *The Turning Point*, London: Flamingo.

Carlen, P. (1988) *Women, Crime and Poverty*, Milton Keynes: Open University Press.

Carse, J., Panton, N. E. and Watt, A. (1958) 'A district mental health service', *Lancet*, 1, 39–41.

Chaika, E. and Lambe, R. A. (1989) 'Cohesion in schizophrenic narratives, revisited', *Journal of Communication Disorders*, 22, 6, 407–21.

Chapell, J. N. and Daniels, R. S. (1970) 'Home visiting in a black urban ghetto', *American Journal of Psychiatry*, 126, 1455–60.

Chapell, J. N. and Daniels, R. S. (1972) 'Home visiting: an aid to psychiatric treatment in a black urban ghettos', *Current Psychiatric Therapies*, 12, 194–201.

Charon, R. (1992) 'To build a case: medical histories as traditions in conflict', *Literature and Medicine*, 11, 1, 115–32.

Chase, S. E. (1995) 'Taking narrative seriously: consequences for method and theory in interview studies', in Josselson, R. and Lieblich, A. (eds) *Interpreting Experience: The Narrative Study of Lives (Volume 3)*, London: Sage.

Chiu, T. L. and Primeau, C. (1991) 'A psychiatric mobile crisis unit in New York City: description and assessment, with implications for mental health care in the 1990s', *International Journal of Social Psychiatry*, 37, 351–8.

Clare, A. (1982) 'Chapter 2', in Shepherd, M. (ed.) *Psychiatrists on Psychiatry*, Cambridge: Cambridge University Press.

Coates, D. B., Kendall, L. M., MaCurdy, E. A. and Goodacre, R. H. (1976) 'Evaluating hospital and home treatment for psychiatric patients', *Canada's Mental Health*, 24, 1, 28–33.

Cohen, B. M. Z. (1996) *Stoned: Changing Police Perceptions of Drugs and Drug Users*, Huddersfield: University of Huddersfield.

Cohen, B. M. Z. (1997a) *Evaluation of The Bradford Home Treatment Service: Interim Report*, Bradford: University of Bradford.

Cohen, B. M. Z. (1997b) *Evaluation of The Bradford Home Treatment Service: Interim Report for Home Treatment Staff Development*, Bradford: University of Bradford.

Cohen, B. M. Z. (1999a) *Evaluation of The Bradford Home Treatment Service: Final Report*, Bradford: University of Bradford.

Cohen, B. M. Z. (1999b) 'Innovatory forms of evaluation for new crisis services', *Science, Discourse and Mind*, 1, 1, 12–31.

Cohen, B. M. Z. (2001) 'Providing intensive home treatment: inter-agency and inter-professional issues', in Brimblecombe, N. (ed.) *Acute Mental Health Care in the Community Intensive Home Treatment*, London: Whurr.

Cohen, D. (1988) *Forgotten Millions: The Treatment of the Mentally Ill – A Global Perspective*, London: Collins.

Cohen, P. S. (1968) *Modern Social Theory*, London: Heinemann.

Coleman, R. (1998) *The Politics of the Madhouse*, Runcorn: Handsell.

Cooper, D. (1967) *Psychiatry and Anti-Psychiatry*, London: Tavistock.

Corin, E. (1990) 'Facts and meaning in psychiatry: An anthropological approach to the lifeworld of schizophrenics', *Culture, Medicine, and Psychiatry*, 14, 2, 153–88.

Critical Psychiatry Network (2000) 'Critical psychiatry', *CPD Bulletin Psychiatry* (online), 2, 33–6, reproduced at http://www.critpsynet.freeuk.com/critical psychiatry.htm (accessed 2 March 2007).

Crossley, N. (1997) *Contesting Psychiatry: Mental Health Movements and Pressure Groups in the Public Sphere in Post-War Britain*, Sheffield: University of Sheffield.

Cuevas-Sosa, A. (2001) 'Postpsychiatry and DSM as a penal code', *British Medical Journal* (online), 24 March, http://www.bmj.com/cgi/eletters/322/7288/724#13442 (accessed 1 March 2007).

Denzin, N. K. (1997) *Interpretative Ethnography: Ethnographic Practices for the 21st Century*, London: Sage.

Department of Health (1998) Frank Dobson Outlines Third Way for Mental Health, press release no. 98/311, 29 July, http://www.dh.gov.uk/Publications-AndStatistics/PressReleases/PressReleasesNotices/fs/en?CONTENT_ID=4024509&chk=G4JMRG (accessed 2 March 2007).

Department of Health (1999) *National Service Framework for Mental Health: Modern Standards and Service Models*, London: Department of Health.

Department of Health (2007) *Mental Health Bill 2006 and the Bill Products Published*, http://www.dh.gov.uk/en/Publicationsandstatistics/DH_063423 (accessed 17 March 2007).

Derrida, J. (1981) *Positions*, Chicago: University of Chicago Press.

Double, D. B. (2005) 'Paradigm shift in psychiatry', in Ramon, S. and Williams, J. (eds) *Mental Health at the Crossroads: The Promise of the Psychosocial Approach* (online), Abingdon: Ashgate, reproduced at http://www.critpsynet.freeuk.com/paradigm.htm (accessed 2 March 2007).

Durkheim, E. (1952) *Suicide: A Study in Sociology*, London: Routledge and Kegan Paul.

Eisenberg, L. (1981) 'The physician as interpreter: ascribing meaning to the illness experience', *Comprehensive Psychiatry*, 22, 239–48.

Elias, N. (1991) *The Society of Individuals*, Oxford: Basil Blackwell.

Estroff, S. E. (1981) *Making It Crazy: Ethnography of Psychiatric Clients in an American Community*, London: University of California Press.

Estroff, S. E., Lachicotte, W. S., Illingworth, L. C. and Johnston, A. (1992) 'Everybody's got a little mental illness: accounts of illness and self among people with severe, persistent mental illness', *Medical Anthropology Quarterly*, 5, 331–69.

European Commission Health and Consumer Protection Directorate-General (2005) *Improving the Mental Health of the Population: Towards a Strategy on Mental Health for the European Union (Green Paper)*, Brussels: European Commission.

Fabrega, H. (1989) 'The self and schizophrenia: a cultural perspective', *Schizophrenia Bulletin*, 15, 2, 277–90.

Fararo, T. J. (1993) 'Generating narrative forms', *Journal of Mathematical Sociology*, 18, 2–3, 153–81.

Faris, R. E. and Dunham, H. W. (1939) *Mental Disorder in Urban Areas: An Ecological Study of Schizophrenia and Other Psychoses*, Chicago: University of Chicago Press.

Fenton, F. R., Tessier, L. and Struening, E. L. (1979) 'A comparative trial of home and hospital psychiatric care', *Archives of General Psychiatry*, 36, 10, 1073–9.

Fenton, F. R., Tessier, L., Struening, E. L., Smith, F. A., Benoit, C. and Contandriopoulos, A. P. (1984) 'A two-year follow-up of a comparative trial of the cost-effectiveness of home and hospital psychiatric treatment', *Canadian Journal of Psychiatry*, 29, 3, 205–11.

Fernando, S. (ed.) (1995) *Mental Health in a Multi-Ethnic Society*, London: Routledge.

Finch, H. L. (1995) *Wittgenstein*, Shaftesbury: Element Books.

Foucault, M. (1967) *Madness and Civilisation: A History of Insanity in the Age of Reason*, London: Routledge.

Foucault, M. (1972) *The Archaeology of Knowledge*, London: Routledge.

Fournaise, V. (1988) 'La psychiatrie de secteur: la visite a domicile en milieu rurale', *Soins Psychiatrie*, 96, 16–18.

Frank, G. (1984) 'Life history model of adaptation to disability', *Social Science and Medicine*, 19, 639–45.

Freeman, H. (1996) '250 years of English psychiatry', *Fortschr Neurol Psychiatr*, 64, 8, 320–6.

Frow, J. and Morris, M. (eds) (1993) *Australian Cultural Studies: A Reader*, Urbana: University of Illinois Press.

Geertz, C. (1983) *Local Knowledge: Further Essays in Interpretative Anthropology*, New York: Basic Books.

Genette, G. (1988) *Narrative Discourse Revisited*, New York: Cornell University Press.

Gergen, K. J. (1994) *Realties and Relationships: Soundings in Social Construction*, Harvard: Harvard University Press.

Gergen, K. J. and Gergen, M. M. (1988) 'Narrative form and the construction of psychological theory', in Sarbin, T. R. (ed.) *The Narrative Perspective in Psychology*, New York: Praeger.

Gergen, K. J. and Kaye, J. (1992) 'Reflection and reconstruction', in McNamee, S. and Goolishian, H. (eds) *Therapy as a Social Construction*, Newbury Park: Sage.

Goffman, E. (1961) *Asylums*, London: Penguin.

Goffman, E. (1963) *Stigma: Notes on the Management of Spoiled Identity*, London: Penguin.

Gomm, R. (1996) 'Mental health and inequality', in Heller, T., Reynolds, J., Gomm, R., Muston, R. and Pattison, S. (eds) *Mental Health Matters: A Reader*, London: Macmillan/Open University Press.

Green, A. E., Maguire, M. and Canny, A. (2001) *Keeping Track: Mapping and Tracking Vulnerable Young People*, Bristol: Policy Press.

Grindrod, J. (1999) 'Goodness gracious Meera', *INK: The Waterstone's Student Magazine*, Autumn, 18–19.

Harré, R. (1993) *Social Being*, 2nd edition, Oxford: Blackwell.

Hart, J. (1992) 'Cracking the code: narrative and political mobilization in the Greek resistance', *Social Science History*, 16, 4, 631–68.

Healthcare Commission (2005) 'Crisis resolution team implementation', http://ratings2005.healthcarecommission.org.uk/Trust/Indicator/IndicatorDescriptionShort.asp?IndicatorId=3202 (accessed 8 March 2007).

Heath, S. B. (1986) 'Taking a cross-cultural look at narratives', *Topics in Language Discourse*, 7, 1, 84–94.

Henry, D. (1999) 'Appropriate or racist?', *Open Mind*, 98, 9.

Herzlich, C. and Pierret, J. (1986) 'Illness: from causes to meaning', in Currer, C. and Stacey, M. (eds) *Concepts of Health, Illness and Disease: A Comparative Perspective*, Oxford: Berg.

Hobbs, M. (1984) 'Crisis intervention in theory and practice: a selective review', *British Journal of Medical Psychology*, 57, 23–34.

Hogan, K. (1997) *The Effectiveness of Crisis Services: A Review of Research*, Paper presented at The 2nd Annual Conference on Crisis Services in Mental Health, Wolverhampton: University of Wolverhampton.

Hogan, K., Crawford-Wright, A., Orme, S., Easthope, Y. and Barker, D. (1997) *Walsall Crisis Support Service Final Report, Volume 2: Literature Review*, Wolverhampton: University of Wolverhampton.

Hollins, S. (2006) 'Talking up the benefits of therapy', *The Guardian* (online), 21 June, http://www.guardian.co.uk/letters/story/0,,1802115,00.html (accessed 2 March 2007).

Horner, E. A. (1995) 'The meeting of two narratives', *Clinical Social Work Journal*, 23, 1, 9–19.

Hoult, J., Reynolds, I., Charbonneau-Powis, M., Weekes, P. and Briggs, J. (1983) 'Psychiatric hospital versus community treatment: the results of a randomised trial', *Australian and New Zealand Journal of Psychiatry*, 17, 160–7.

Ingleby, D. (1981) 'Understanding "mental illness" ', in Ingleby, D. (ed.) *Critical Psychiatry: The Politics of Mental Health*, Harmondsworth: Penguin.

James, A. (2000) 'New mentality', *The Guardian* (online), 26 January, http://society.guardian.co.uk/societyguardian/story/0,7843,391194,00.html (accessed 19 February 2007).

James, A. (2006) 'Government drops key proposals of draft Mental Health Bill', *Psychminded.co.uk* (online), 23 March, http://www.psychminded.co.uk/news/news2006/march06/Government%20drops%20key%20proposals.htm (accessed 9 February 2007).

Jané-Llopis, E. and Anderson, P. (2005) *Mental Health Promotion and Mental Disorder Prevention: A Policy for Europe*, Nijmegen: Radboud University Nijmegen.

Jenkins, J. H. (1988) 'Conceptions of schizophrenia as a problem of nerves: a cross-cultural comparison of Mexican-Americans and Anglo-Americans', *Social Science and Medicine*, 26, 12, 1233–43.

Jervis, G. (1975) *Manuale Critico di Psichiatrica*, Milano: Feltrinelli.

Jodelet, D. (1991) *Madness and Social Representations*, London: Harvester Wheatsheaf.

Johnstone, L. (1989) *User and Abusers of Psychiatry*, London: Routledge.

Josselson, R. (1995) 'Imagining the real: empathy, narrative, and the dialogic self', in Josselson, R. and Lieblich, A. (eds) *Interpreting Experience: The Narrative Study of Lives (Volume 3)*, London: Sage.

Josselson, R. and Lieblich, A. (eds) (1993) *The Narrative Study of Lives (Volume 1)*, London: Sage.

Josselson, R. and Lieblich, A. (eds) (1995a) *Interpreting Experience: The Narrative Study of Lives (Volume 3)*, London: Sage.

Josselson, R. and Lieblich, A. (1995b) 'Introduction', in Josselson, R. and Lieblich, A. (eds) *Interpreting Experience: The Narrative Study of Lives (Volume 3)*, London: Sage.

Kaufman, S. R. (1988) 'Toward a phenomenology of boundaries in medicine: chronic illness experience in the case of stroke', *Medical Anthropology Quarterly*, 2, NS, 338–54.

Kirmayer, L. J. (1992) 'The body's insistence on meaning: metaphor as presentation and representation in illness experience', *Medical Anthropology Quarterly*, 6, 4, 323–46.

Kleinman, A. (1986) 'Concepts and a model for the comparison of medical systems as cultural systems', in Currer, C. and Stacey, M. (eds) *Concepts of Health, Illness and Disease: A Comparative Perspective*, Oxford: Berg.

Kleinman, A. (1988) *The Illness Narratives: Suffering, Healing and the Human Condition*, London: Harper Collins.

Kleinman, A. and Good, B. J. (eds) (1985) *Culture and Depression*, Berkeley: University of California Press.

Korchin, S. J. (1976) *Modern Clinical Psychology: Principles of Interpretation in the Clinic and the Community*, New York: Harper & Row.

Kosky, R. (1986) 'From morality to madness: a reappraisal of the asylum movement in psychiatry 1800–1940', *Australian and New Zealand Journal of Psychiatry*, 20, 180–7.

Kroll, J. and Bachrach, B. (1984) 'Sin and mental illness in the Middle Ages', *Psychological Medicine*, 14, 507–14.

Lapsley, H., Waimarie Nikora, L. and Black, R. (2002) *'Kia Mauri Tau!': Narratives of Recovery from Disabling Mental Health Problems*, Wellington: Mental Health Commission.

Ledwith, F., Husband, C. and Karmani, A. (1997) *Promoting Inter-Agency Mental Health Provision for Ethnic Minorities*, Bradford: University of Bradford Ethnicity & Social Policy Research Unit.

Lee, R. E. and Dwyer, T. (1995) 'Co-constructed narratives around being "sick": a minimalist model', *Contemporary Family Therapy*, 17, 1, 65–82.

Lin, K. M. and Kleinman, A. R. (1988) 'Psychopathology and clinical course of schizophrenia: A cross-cultural perspective', *Schizophrenia Bulletin*, 14, 4, 555–67.

Lyotard, J. F. (1979) *The Post-Modern Condition: A Report on Knowledge*, Manchester: Manchester University Press.

MacMillan, D. (1958) 'Mental health services in Nottingham', *International Journal of Social Psychiatry*, 4, 5–9.

Marcus, G. E. (1994) 'What comes (just) after the 'post'? The case of ethnography', in Denzin, N. K. and Lincoln, Y. S. (eds) *The Handbook of Qualitative Research*, California: Sage.

Marks, I. M., Connolly, J. and Muijen, M. (1988) 'The Maudsley daily living programme: a controlled cost-effectiveness study of community-based versus standard in-patient care of serious mental illness', *Bulletin of the Royal College of Psychiatrists*, 12, 22–3.

Marks, I. M., Connolly, J., Muijen, M., Audini, B., McNamee, G. and Lawrence, R. E. (1994) 'Home-based versus hospital-based care for people with serious mental illness', *British Journal of Psychiatry*, 165, 179–94.

Masson, J. (1989) *Against Therapy*, London: Collins.

Mattingly, C. (1991) 'The narrative nature of clinical reasoning', *American Journal of Occupational Therapy*, 45, 998–1005.

Mattingly, C. and Garro, L. C. (1994) 'Introduction', *Social Science Medicine*, 38, 6, 771–4.

Maurin, F. (1990) 'Pratique d'infirmier "aux visites a domicile" du secteur 12', *Soins Psichiatrie*, 110/111, 45–8.

Maynes, M. J. (1992) 'Autobiography and class formation in nineteenth-century Europe: Methodological considerations', *Social Science History*, 16, 3, 517–37.

McLaughlin, K. (2006) 'Scare in the community', *Spiked* (online), 6 December, http://www.spiked-online.com/index.php?/site/article/2212 (accessed 17 March 2007).

Melichar, J. K. and Argyropoulos, S. V. (2001) '"Postpsychiatry" – or merely "Properly Funded Psychiatry"?', *British Medical Journal* (online), 24 March, http://www.bmj.com/cgi/eletters/322/7288/724#13441 (accessed 1 March 2007).

Merton, R. K. (1957) *Social Theory and Social Structure*, Glencoe: Free Press.

Meyer, R. E., Schiff, L. F. and Becker, A. (1967) 'The home treatment of psychotic patients: an analysis of 154 cases', *American Journal of Psychiatry*, 123, 1430–8.

Michaelson-Kanfer, A. (1993) 'Some comments on some aspects of comparative narratives', *Journal of Mathematical Sociology*, 18, 2–3, 215–7.

Mickle, J. C. (1963) 'Psychiatric home visits', *Archives of General Psychiatry*, 9, 91–5.

Miller, B. (2006) 'Ban ECT and junk the drugs. And whatever you do, don't follow the US example. Peter Breggin spells it out', http://wellbeingfoundation.com/interviews_pg1.html (accessed 5 March 2007).

Miller, P. (1986) 'Critiques of psychiatry and critical sociologies of madness', in Miller, P. and Rose, N. (eds) *The Power of Psychiatry*, Cambridge: Polity.

Miller, S. G. (1994) 'Borderline personality disorder from the patient's perspective', *Hospital and Community Psychiatry*, 45, 12, 1215–19.

Miller, W. B. (1958), 'Lower class culture as a generating milieu of gang delinquency', *Journal of Social Issues*, 14, 3, 5–19.

MIND (2003) *Mind Seminar Discusses Urgent Mental Health Needs of Black and Ethnic Minorities in the Run up to Government Report*, press release, 6 March, http://www.mind.org.uk/News+policy+and+campaigns/Press+archive/Mind+seminar+discusses+urgent+mental+health+needs+of+black+and+ethnic+minorities+in+the+run+up+to+go.htm (accessed 25 March 2007).

MIND (2005) 'Statistics 1: How common is mental distress?' http://www.mind.org.uk/Information/Factsheets/Statistics/Statistics+1.htm#How%20many%20people%20in%20Britain%20experience%20mental%20health%20problems? (accessed 16 March 2007).

MIND (2006) 'Dangerousness and mental health: the facts', http://www.mind.org.uk/Information/Factsheets/Dangerousness.htm (accessed 17 March 2007).

MIND (2007a) *Care Before Compulsion Best Route to Reduce Risk, Says Mind*, press release, http://www.mind.org.uk/News+policy+and+campaigns/Press/2006-09-15+DH+Risk+Management+Programme.htm (accessed 16 March 2007).

MIND (2007b) 'Factsheets and booklets by subject: drugs', http://www.mind.org.uk/Information/Factsheets/#D (accessed 22 March 2007).

Mitchell, J. C. (ed.) (1969) *Social Networks in Urban Situations*, Manchester: Manchester University Press.

Moncrieff, J. (2003) *Is Psychiatry for Sale? An Examination of the Influence of the Pharmaceutical Industry on Academic and Practical Psychiatry*, Maudsley discussion paper, London: Institute of Psychiatry.

Moncrieff, J., Hopker, S. and Thomas, P. (2005) 'Psychiatry and the pharmaceutical industry: who pays the piper? A perspective from the Critical Psychiatry Network', *Psychiatric Bulletin*, 29, 84–5.

Mosher, L. R., Menn, A. and Matthew, S. M. (1975) 'Soteria: evaluation of a home-based treatment for schizophrenia', *American Journal of Orthopsychiatry*, 45, 3, 455–67.

Moynihan, R. and Cassels, A. (2005) *Selling Sickness: How Drug Companies are Turning us all into Patients*, Crows Nest: Allen & Unwin.

Muijen, M. (1996) 'Scare in the community: Britain in moral panic', in Heller, T., Reynolds, J., Gomm, R., Muston, R. and Pattison, S. (eds) *Mental Health Matters: A Reader*, London: Macmillan/Open University Press.

Muijen, M., Marks, I., Connolly, J. and Audini, B. (1992) 'Home based care and standard hospital care for patients with severe mental illness: A randomised controlled trail', *British Medical Journal*, 304, 749–54.

Murphy, R. M. (1989) *The Body Silent*, New York: Holt.

Nash, C. (1990) 'Forward', in Nash, C. (ed.) *Narrative in Culture*, London: Routledge.

National Health Service (2002) 'Mental health beacon: Bradford Home Treatment Service', http://www.nyx.org.uk/beacons/mental/bradfordhome.htm (accessed 19 February 2007).

Newton, S. (1989) 'Organisational models for crisis intervention', in Renshaw, J. (ed.) *Crisis Intervention Services Information Pack*, London: Good Practices in Mental Health.

Norris, C. (1987) *Derrida*, London: Harper Collins.

Office for National Statistics (2001) *Mental Health Among Adults*, press release, 18 December, http://www.statistics.gov.uk/pdfdir/mhaa1201.pdf (accessed 13 March 2007).

Orme, S. and Cohen, B. M. Z. (2001) 'Researching services providing IHT as an alternative to admission', in Brimblecombe, N. (ed.) *Acute Mental Health Care in the Community: Intensive Home Treatment*, London: Whurr.

Palombo, J. (1992) 'Narratives, self-cohesion, and the patient's search for meaning', *Clinical Social Work Journal*, 20, 3, 249–70.

Parker, I. (ed.) (1999) *Deconstructing Psychotherapy*, London: Sage.

Parsons, T. (1937) *The Structure of Social Action*, New York: Free Press.

Peay, J. (ed.) (1996) *Inquiries after Homicide*, London: Duckworth.

Peloquin, S. M. (1993) 'The depersonalization of patients: a profile gleamed from narratives', *American Journal of Occupational Therapy*, 47, 9, 830–7.

Perring, C. (1992) 'The experience and perspectives of patients and care staff of the transition from hospital to community-based care', in Ramon, S. (ed.) *Psychiatric Hospital Closure: Myths and Realities*, London: Chapman & Hall.

Pilgrim, D. (1999) 'Badly in need of help', *Open Mind*, 95, 7.

Pilgrim, D. and Rogers, A. (1996) 'Two notions of risk in mental health debates', in Heller, T., Reynolds, J., Gomm, R., Muston, R. and Pattison, S. (eds) *Mental Health Matters: A Reader*, London: Macmillan/Open University Press.

Pill, R. and Stott, N. (1986) 'Concepts of illness causation and responsibility: some preliminary data from a sample of working-class mothers', in Currer, C. and Stacey, M. (eds) *Concepts of Health, Illness and Disease: A Comparative Perspective*, Oxford: Berg.

Plummer, K. (1983) *Documents of Life*, London: George Allen & Unwin.

Polakk, P. R. and Kirby, M. W. (1976) 'A model to replace psychiatric hospitals', *The Journal of Nervous and Mental Disease*, 162, 1, 13–22.

President's New Freedom Commission on Mental Health (2003) *Achieving the Promise: Transforming Mental Health Care in America*, Rockville: Substance Abuse and Mental Health Services Administration.

Prior, L. (1993) *The Social Organisation of Mental Illness*, London: Sage.

Psychology Politics Resistance (1998) *Newsletter No.5*, Bolton: Bolton Institute.

Querido, A. (1968) 'The shaping of community mental health care', *British Journal of Psychiatry*, 114, 293–302.

Ramon, S. (1996) *Mental Health in Europe: Ends, Beginnings and Rediscoveries*, London: Macmillan.

Ranjith, G. and Mohan, R. (2001) 'Postpsychiatry and antipsychiatry: old wine in new bottles', *British Medical Journal* (online), 27 March, http://www.bmj.com/cgi/eletters/322/7288/724#13524 (accessed 1 March 2007).

Rapley, M. (2001) 'Postpsychiatry and critical psychology', *British Medical Journal* (online), 28 March, http://www.bmj.com/cgi/eletters/322/7288/724#13545 (accessed 1 March 2007).

Read, J. and Reynolds, J. (eds) (1996) *Speaking Our Minds: An Anthology of Personal Experiences of Mental Distress and its Consequences*, London: Macmillan.

Reid, H. (1989) 'Hospitalized psychiatry', in Brackx, A. and Grimshaw, C. (eds) *Mental Health Care in Crisis*, London: Pluto.

Relton, P. and Thomas, P. (2002) 'Alternatives to acute wards: users' perspectives', *Psychiatric Bulletin*, 26, 346–7.

Renshaw, J. (1989) 'Crisis intervention: introduction', in Renshaw, J. (ed.) *Crisis Intervention Services Information Pack*, London: Good Practices in Mental Health.

Rosaldo, R. (1989) *Culture and Truth*, Boston: Beacon.

Rose, N. (1989) *Governing the Soul: The Shaping of the Private Self*, London: Routledge.

Rose, N. (1999) *Governing the Soul: The Shaping of the Private Self*, 2nd edition, London: Free Association Books.

Rosenau, P. M. (1992) *Post-Modernism and the Social Sciences: Insights, Inroads, and Intrusions*, Chichester: Princeton University Press.

Rosenhan, D. L. (1996) 'On being sane in insane places', in Heller, T., Reynolds, J., Gomm, R., Muston, R. and Pattison, S. (eds) *Mental Health Matters: A Reader*, London: Macmillan/Open University Press.

Rosenzweig, A., Pasternak, R., Booth, B., Morycz, R., Fox, A., Hoch, C. and Reynolds, C. (1996) 'In-home psychiatric treatment of elderly patients: descriptive characteristics and outcome measures', *The American Journal of Geriatric Psychiatry*, 4, 4, 351.

Russell, B. (1984) *A History of Western Philosophy*, London: Unwin.

Saari, C. (1991) *The Creation of Meaning in Clinical Social Work*, New York: The Guilford Press.

Samson, C. (1995a) 'The fracturing of medical dominance in British psychiatry?', *Sociology of Health and Illness*, 17, 2, 245–68.

Samson, C. (1995b) 'Madness and psychiatry', in Turner, B. S. (ed.) *Medical Power and Social Knowledge*, 2nd edition, London: Sage.

Saris, A. J. (1995) 'Telling stories: life histories, illness narratives, and institutional landscapes', *Culture, Medicine and Psychiatry*, 19, 39–72.

Sashidharan, S. P. and Smyth, M. (1992) *Evaluation of Home Treatment in Ladywood: Results from the First Two Years*, Birmingham: North Birmingham Home Treatment Service.
Scheff, T. J. (1996) 'Labelling mental illness', in Heller, T., Reynolds, J., Gomm, R., Muston, R. and Pattison, S. (eds) *Mental Health Matters: A Reader*, London: Macmillan/Open University Press.
Schutz, A. (1962) 'Commonsense and scientific interpretation of human action', in Schutz, A. (ed.) *Collected Papers Volume 1*, The Hague: Martinus Nijhoff.
Scull, A. (1981a) 'Introduction', in Scull, A. (ed.) *Madhouses, Mad-Doctors and Madmen: The Social History of Psychiatry in the Victorian Era*, London: The Athlone Press.
Scull, A. (1981b) 'Moral treatment reconsidered: some sociological comments on an episode in the history of British psychiatry', in Scull, A. (ed.) *Madhouses, Mad-Doctors and Madmen: The Social History of Psychiatry in the Victorian Era*, London: The Athlone Press.
Scull, A. (1984) *Decarceration: Community Treatment and the Deviant – A Radical View*, 2nd edition, Oxford: Basil Blackwell.
Sedgwick, P. (1982) *Psycho Politics*, London: Pluto Press.
Seelig, W. R., Goldman-Hall, B. J. and Jerrell, J. M. (1992) 'In-home treatment of families with seriously disturbed adolescents in crisis', *Family Process*, 31, 2, 135–49.
Sewell, W. H. (1992) 'Introduction: narrative and social identities', *Social Science History*, 16, 3, 479–88.
Shepherd, M. (1966) *Psychiatric Illness in General Practice*, London: Oxford University Press.
Shotter, J. (1989) 'Social accountability and the social construction of "you" ', in Shotter, J. and Gergen, K. J. (eds) *Texts of Identity*, London: Sage.
Showalter, E. (1992) 'On hysterical narrative', *Narrative*, 1, 24–35.
Sims, A. (1989) 'What is the role of the consultant in the community?', *Psychiatric Bulletin*, 13, 285–7.
Singer, J. A. (1995) 'Putting emotion in context: it's place within individual and social narratives', *Journal of Narrative and Life History*, 5, 3, 255–67.
Singer, P., Holloway, B. and Kolb, L. C. (1969) 'The psychiatrist-nurse team and home care in the Soviet Union and Amsterdam', *American Journal of Psychiatry*, 125, 1198–202.
Slater, E. and Roth, M. (1969) *Clinical Psychiatry*, 2nd edition, London: Balliere, Tindall and Cassell.
Smart, B. (1985) *Michel Foucault*, London: Ellis Horwood and Tavistock.
Smith, D. E. (1978) ' "K is mentally ill": the anatomy of a factual account', *Sociology*, 12, 1, 23–53.
Smith, M. (1997) 'Role of the popular media in mental illness', *The Lancet*, 349, 1779.
Smith, S. (2001) 'Is postpsychiatry so radical?', *British Medical Journal* (online), 3 May, http://www.bmj.com/cgi/eletters/322/7288/724#14144 (accessed 1 March 2007).
Smyth, M. G. and Hoult, J. (2000) 'The home treatment enigma', *British Medical Journal* (online), 320, 305–9, http://www.bmj.com/cgi/content/full/320/7230/305 (accessed 19 February 2007).
Spence, D. (1982) *Narrative Truth and Historical Truth: Meaning and Interpretation in Psychoanalysis*, New York: Norton.

Steinmetz, G. (1992) 'Reflections on the role of social narrative in working-class formation: narrative theory in the social sciences', *Social Science History*, 16, 3, 489–516.

Stern, D. N. (1985) *The Interpersonal World of the Infant*, New York: Basic Books.

Stevens, S. S. (1976) 'Operationism and logical positivism', in Marx, M. H. and Goodson, F. E. (eds) *Theories in Contemporary Psychology*, 2nd edition, New York: Macmillan.

Sundberg, N. D., Taplin, J. R. and Tyler, L. E. (1983) *Introduction to Clinical Psychology: Perspectives, Issues and Contributions to Human Service*, Englewood Cliffs: Prentice Hall.

Surgerydoor (2002) ' "Crisis resolution" teams for mentally ill', 2 January, http://www.surgerydoor.co.uk/news/detail.asp?offset=1677 (accessed 23 February 2007).

Susko, M. A. (1994) 'Caseness and narrative: contrasting approaches to people who are psychiatrically labelled', *The Journal of Mind and Behaviour*, 15, 1–2, 87–112.

Szasz, T. S. (1970) *Ideology and Insanity: Essays on the Psychiatric Dehumanization of Man*, Harmondsworth: Penguin.

Szasz, T. S. (1971) *The Manufacture of Madness*, London: Routledge & Kegan Paul.

Taylor, A. J. W., Robinson, R. D. and McCormick, I. A. (1986) 'Written personal narratives as research documents – The case for their restoration', *International Review of Applied Psychology*, 35, 2, 197–208.

Test, M. A. and Stein, L. I. (1980) 'Alternatives to mental hospital treatment III: social costs', *Archives of General Psychiatry*, 37, 409–12.

Thompson, E. P. (1972) 'Anthropology and the discipline of historical context', *Midland History*, 1, 3, 41–55.

Thompson, P. (1978) *The Voice of the Past: Oral History*, Oxford: Oxford University Press.

Thornicroft, G. and Tansella, M. (2004) 'Components of a modern mental health service: a pragmatic balance of community and hospital care', *British Journal of Psychiatry*, 185, 283–90.

Tufnell, G., Bouras, N., Watson, J. P. and Brough, D. I. (1985) 'Home assessment and treatment in a community psychiatric service', *Acta Psychiatrica Scandinavica*, 72, 1, 20–8.

Turner, B. S. (1987) *Medical Power and Social Knowledge*, London: Sage.

Turner, B. S. (1995) *Medical Power and Social Knowledge*, 2nd edition, London: Sage.

Tyrer, P., Turner, R. and Johnson, A. L. (1989) 'Integrated hospital and community psychiatric services and use of inpatient beds', *British Medical Journal*, 299, 298–300.

United States Department of Health and Human Services (2002) *Mental Health Topics: Mental Illnesses/Disorders*, http://mentalhealth.samhsa.gov/topics/explore/mentalillness (accessed 13 March 2007).

Weber, M. (1958) *The Protestant Ethic and the Spirit of Capitalism*, New York: Charles Scribner's Sons.

Wilson, M. (1999) 'Cautious optimism', *Open Mind*, 98, 7.

Wing, J. K., Bebbington, P. and Robins, L. N. (1981) *What is a Case? The Problem of Definition in Psychiatric Community Surveys*, London: Grant McIntyre.

Woof, K., Goldberg, D. and Fryers, T. (1988) 'The practice of community psychiatric nursing and mental health social work in Salford: some implications for community care', *British Journal of Psychiatry*, 152, 783–92.

World Health Organization (2005a) 'Glaring inequalities for people with mental disorders addressed in new WHO effort', http://www.who.int/mediacentre/news/notes/2005/np14/en/index.html (accessed 13 March 2007).

World Health Organization (2005b) 'New WHO mental health atlas shows global mental health resources remain inadequate', http://www.who.int/mediacentre/news/notes/2005/np21/en/index.html (accessed 13 March 2007).

Zohar, A. H. (1995) 'Developmental patterns of mathematically gifted individuals as viewed through their narratives', in Josselson, R. and Lieblich, A. (eds) *Interpreting Experience: The Narrative Study of Lives (Volume 3)*, London: Sage.

Zola, I. K. (ed.) (1982) *Ordinary Lives: Voices of Disability and Disease*, Cambridge: Applewood Books.

Zukier, H. (1986) 'The paradigmatic and narrative modes in goal-guided inference', in Sorrentino, R. M. and Higgins, E. T. (eds) *Handbook of Motivation and Cognition*, New York: Guildford.

Zweig, S. (1979) *Erasmus, and the Right to Heresy*, London: Souvenir Press.

Index

GPSR Compliance
The European Union's (EU) General Product Safety Regulation (GPSR) is a set of rules that requires consumer products to be safe and our obligations to ensure this.

If you have any concerns about our products, you can contact us on

ProductSafety@springernature.com

In case Publisher is established outside the EU, the EU authorized representative is:

Springer Nature Customer Service Center GmbH
Europaplatz 3
69115 Heidelberg, Germany

www.ingramcontent.com/pod-product-compliance
Ingram Content Group UK Ltd.
Pitfield, Milton Keynes, MK11 3LW, UK
UKHW020043040925
462575UK00013B/515
* 9 7 8 1 3 4 9 5 2 2 9 7 2 *